PATIENT-CENTERED PROGNOSIS: A METHODOLOGY TO IMPROVE INDIVIDUALLY
TAILORED PROGNOSTIC ACCURACY ILLUSTRATED IN TWO CANCERS

James R. Miller III, PhD
Mohammed Kashani-Sabet, MD
Richard W. Sagebiel, MD

April 2013

iUniverse LLC
Bloomington

PATIENT-CENTERED PROGNOSIS: A METHODOLOGY TO IMPROVE INDIVIDUALLY
TAILORED PROGNOSTIC ACCURACY ILLUSTRATED IN TWO CANCERS

iUniverse books may be ordered through booksellers or by contacting:

iUniverse
1663 Liberty Drive
Bloomington, IN 47403
www.iuniverse.com
1-800-Authors (1-800-288-4677)

ISBN: 978-1-4917-0680-0 (sc)
ISBN: 978-1-4917-0681-7 (e)

Library of Congress Control Number: 2013916238

Printed in the United States of America.

iUniverse rev. date: 10/7/2013

CONTENTS

                                                                        Page

PREFACE iv

ACKNOWLEDGEMENTS vi

1.0 INTRODUCTION 1

     1.1 A Ten-Step Individually Tailored Prognostic Methodology 1
     1.2 An Historical Trigger 4
     1.3 How PCM Differs from Traditional Prognostic Methodology 5

2.0 RECONSTRUCTING CURRENT PROGNOSTIC METHODOLOGY 10

     2.1 Selecting a Focal End Point 10
     2.2 Selecting Individually Tailored Measures to Calibrate
          Prognostic Accuracy 12
     2.3 Establishing a Base Case for Assessing Accuracy Improvements .. 14
     2.4 Stratifying Patients According to Risk of Experiencing the
          Focal Event 16
     2.5 Admissibility Requirements for Traditional and Nontraditional
          Factors 17
     2.6 Partitioning Each Factor Scale to Optimize Univariate
          Discriminability 18
     2.7 Assigning Impact-Reflecting Index Values to Partitioned Factor
          Subscales 21
     2.8 Weighting Impact-Reflecting Index (UIRI) Values across
          Prognostic Factors 24
     2.9 Merging Separate Risk Groups and Incorporating Nontraditional
          Factors 25
     2.10 Statistical Consequences of an Altered Focus and Novel Success
          Measures 27

3.0 APPLYING PCM TO 1,222 MELANOMA PATIENTS 31

     3.1 Stratifying Patients into Low-Risk, Medium-Risk, and High-Risk
          Subgroups 32
     3.2 Analysis of Traditional Prognostic Factors without Missing
          Observations 34
     3.3 Analysis of Traditional Prognostic Factors with Missing
          Observations 40
     3.4 Adding Nontraditional Prognostic Factors to the Analysis 51
     3.5 Summary of Melanoma Results 52
     3.6 Applying Tailored Individual Probabilities to Making
          Therapeutic Choices 59

4.0 APPLYING PCM TO 1,225 BREAST CANCER PATIENTS 63

    4.1 Stratifying Patients into Low-Risk, Medium-Risk, and High-Risk
         Subgroups 63

    4.2 Analysis of Traditional Prognostic Factors without Missing
         Observations 65

    4.3 Analysis of Traditional Prognostic Factors with Missing
         Observations 71

    4.4 Adding Nontraditional Prognostic Factors to the Analysis 79

    4.5 How Selection Bias Can Severely Distort the Apparent Efficacy
         of Therapy 80

    4.6 Summary of Breast Cancer Results 83

5.0 CONCLUSIONS AND RECOMMENDATIONS 90

APPENDIXES 103

    Appendix A - A Simplified Illustration and Assessment of the
    Patient-Centered Methodology 103

    Appendix B - Attributes of the 1,222 Patients Included within the
    Melanoma Training Sample 130

    Appendix C - Relative Prognostic Weights in Differentiating the
    Incidence of MM DEATH=<5YRS Generated by Least-Squares Weighting
    Rescaled Univariate Impact Probabilities 138

    Appendix D - Attributes of the 1,225 Patients Included within the
    Breast Cancer Training Sample 141

    Appendix E - Relative Prognostic Weights in Differentiating the
    Incidence of MBC DEATH=<5YRS Generated by Least-Squares Weighting
    Rescaled Univariate Impact Probabilities 148

    Appendix F - Two Limited-Scope, Split-Sample Reliability Analyses
    Designed to Replicate and Validate PCM's Superior Predictive
    Accuracy 152

ANNOTATED REFERENCES 163

INDEX 165

PREFACE

The practice of medicine is both an art and a science.

Underlying the practice of medicine as an art is the clear recognition that no two human beings are exactly alike. Diagnosis, prognosis, and treatment selection decisions cannot be carried out as if individual differences did not exist. They abound. Even identical twins gradually develop small differences in their DNA due to different mutations relating to their separate life paths.

It therefore makes sense to practice medicine in an experience-based manner. A physician's personal experience frequently provides a sensitive and effective guide to tailoring medical care to individual patient needs. The many and varied dissimilarities between individual patient personalities, their cultural and religious backgrounds, and their unique life situations render sole reliance on scientific generalities quite inappropriate.

Underlying the practice of medicine as a science is the equally clear recognition that human beings constitute a particular biological species. Most of us have a single head, two arms, and two legs; a single heart, two separate kidneys, and a brain with two separate, but highly interconnected hemispheres; and so forth. These regularities amply justify treating medicine as a science.

It therefore also makes sense to practice medicine in an evidence-based manner. The collective experience of many physicians is typically superior to that of any single physician. We can exploit what we come to know as common among many or most human beings if we collect patient data and organize our medical practice in a systematic, scientific manner.

Prognostic research in medicine seeks to identify useful indicators of a patient's future state of health.

An indicator is called a prognostic factor when it can be shown to influence salient patient outcomes, such as the future course of cancer and other progressive diseases. Explaining the exact manner in which an underlying factor exerts its influence is an important goal of prognostic research.

An indicator is also prognostically useful if it merely predicts salient patient outcomes. This can happen even without understanding the exact nature of its biological linking mechanisms and pathways. For example, the size of a primary tumor in the initial diagnosis of colorectal cancer, breast cancer, and melanoma matters. Smaller tumors generally portend more favorable patient outcomes. The reasons for this predictive relationship are substantially, but not fully understood. Only its existence and direction seem completely clear. A similar distinction can be drawn between understanding in detail the mechanisms and pathways linking newly discovered biomarkers to disease outcomes (e.g., the biological role of particular genes) and using what limited knowledge we have about biomarkers to make simple, directional predictions.

Prognostic research that focuses primarily on the underlying factors influencing salient patient outcomes we shall characterize as factor-centered. Patients are viewed as carriers of these underlying factors and their salient outcomes. Detailed (sometimes quantitative) models are constructed to connect factors and outcomes. Research conclusions are about the factors. They describe common linkage pathways and associated mechanisms, but not particular patients.

Prognostic research that focuses primarily on making separate, individually tailored predictions of salient patient outcomes we shall characterize as patient-centered. Prognostic factors serve mainly as the basis for making individually tailored predictions. Research conclusions are based on at least a partial understanding of underlying mechanisms and pathways, but they apply separately to each individual patient.

The flavor of factor-centered prognostic research is perhaps more comfortably allied with viewing medicine as a science. The flavor of patient-centered prognostic research is perhaps more comfortably allied with viewing medicine as an art.

However, a central thesis of this book is that the two flavors are completely complementary. Traditional methodology developed in the service of factor-centered research is essential to making predictions of individual patient outcomes, but the accuracy of such predictions can be improved by modifying traditional methodology in certain selective ways. Simultaneously, some, but not all of these selective modifications are useful in drawing traditional, factor-centered conclusions.

Our book is about patient-centered prognosis and how to make individually tailored patient predictions more accurate. The authors have spent the last several decades at the University of California San Francisco (UCSF) and at the California Pacific Medical Center (CPMC) both caring for melanoma patients and producing, collecting, and verifying their medical records. These medical records are used to demonstrate improvements in predictive accuracy realizable by implementing the selective modifications that constitute our patient-centered methodology.

Medical records of breast cancer patients were collected in Finland between 1945 and 1996. These records are also used to demonstrate similar improvements in predictive accuracy realizable by applying our patient-centered methodology to a different cancer and a different patient population.

The results reported and the conclusions drawn in this book are promising, but not definitive. We hope to encourage some centralized organization with significant resources to replicate, if possible, the improvements in predictive accuracy that our patient-centered methodology appears to offer. This means selecting a particular progressive disease, such as a specific cancer, and launching a large-scale replication project. It is not unlike the situation where promising results have been achieved in phase I and phase II clinical trials and the next step is to achieve definitive results in phase III.

ACKNOWLEDGEMENTS

The melanoma data set was produced, collected, verified, and corrected largely by the three authors at the University of California San Francisco (UCSF) during the last four decades. Many additional UCSF personnel provided able assistance in this activity. Particularly noteworthy among the many other UCSF contributors were Dr. Stanley Leong, MD, and Mehdi Nosrati, BS.

Research access to the breast cancer data set collected in Turku, Finland, was granted in April 1999. It was understood that these data would only be used for research purposes and that those involved in collecting and maintaining the data would be properly acknowledged.

The Turku data were carefully collected, regularly checked, and painstakingly updated over a fifty-one-year period between 1945 and 1996. It is largely because of the cleanliness of the data and the duration and thoroughness of patient follow-up that the Finnish data were used, along with the UCSF data, to illustrate the methodology described in this book. The authors are indebted to Dr. Johan Lundin, MD, PhD, and to Dr. Michael Lundin, MD, both of the HUCH Clinical Research Institute, Helsinki, Finland. They transmitted the Turku data set to us in 1999.

The authors are likewise indebted to Dr. Harry B. Burke, MD, PhD, then Associate Professor of Medicine, George Washington University School of Medicine, Washington D. C. It was through his association with the doctors in Finland that the Finnish data set was obtained in April 1999. Both Dr. Burke and one of the authors served at that time as part-time consultants to the Breast Care Center at UCSF, headed by Dr. Laura Esserman, MD, MBA. The authors are especially indebted to Dr. Esserman and to Dr. Debu Tripathy, MD, for their important role in seeking and obtaining the Finnish data.

Critical to achieving the results reported in this book were the efforts of Dr. Heikki Joensuu, MD, then from the Departments of Oncology and Radiotherapy, and Pathology, University Central Hospital of Turku, Turku, Finland, and of Dr. Sakari Toikkanen, MD, then from the Department of Radiotherapy and Oncology, University of Helsinki, Helsinki, Finland. They ensured the cleanliness of the Finnish data. Their initial analysis of the Turku data set was published in a 1995 article in the *Journal of Clinical Oncology* entitled "Cured of Breast Cancer?".

Dr. Joensuu recently joined with the three authors of this book in coauthoring "A Patient-Centered Methodology That Improves the Accuracy of Prognostic Predictions in Cancer" published online by *PLoS One*, February 2013.

Special thanks are due to Mehdi Nosrati, BS, currently at the California Pacific Medical Center Research Institute, for producing the sixteen figures presented in this book.

PATIENT-CENTERED PROGNOSIS: A METHODOLOGY TO IMPROVE INDIVIDUALLY
TAILORED PROGNOSTIC ACCURACY ILLUSTRATED IN TWO CANCERS

1.0   INTRODUCTION

A Patient-Centered Methodology (PCM) has been designed to improve the accuracy
of individually tailored prognoses in dealing with cancer patients. The same
methodology may improve the accuracy of individual patient prognoses in other
progressive diseases, such as diabetes, multiple sclerosis, and heart disease.
It might also be useful relative to nonprogressive diseases and in various
nonmedical contexts.

What does it mean for a prognostic methodology to be "patient-centered"? The
answer, of course, lies in "patient-centered compared to what?" Let us begin by
distinguishing between becoming patient-centered in making focused predictions
of patient outcomes and remaining prognostic factor-centered. The
factor-centered approach is the currently established paradigm in prognostic
research. Based both on its historical success and on its role as a necessary
precursor to becoming patient-centered, this is a fortunate state of affairs.

Becoming patient-centered is a natural extension of already being
factor-centered. It constitutes an enhancement to an existing methodological
orientation rather than an alternative orientation. One cannot become
effectively patient-centered without having first achieved substantial
factor-centered success.

Both the factor-centered and the patient-centered methodological orientations
are being viewed here from an evidence-based perspective. This is not to deny
the efficacy of alternative approaches. For example, a faith-based treatment
protocol may well prove quite beneficial in many ways to many patients
suffering from various forms of cancer. However, only prognostic methodologies
based on empirical medical evidence will be discussed and compared.

1.1   A Ten-Step Individually Tailored Prognostic Methodology

If individually tailored patient prognoses are to be evidence-based, one may:

1. begin with a targeted individual patient, and choose some salient
   state, event, situation or outcome as the focal end point of interest;
2. identify a group of patients similar to the targeted patient in certain
   respects that are relevant to predicting that patient's focal end
   point;
3. identify a set of prognostic factors that can be demonstrated to be
   useful in predicting the focal end point within the specific group
   identified as similar patients;
4. gather observations on these prognostic factors from a sample of these
   similar patients (henceforth referred to as the training data);
5. pick a prognostic model (e.g., a regression model) that predicts the
   focal end point based on each patient's prognostic factor observations;
6. use the sample data to train the model—to estimate via an appropriate
   statistical technique (e.g., likelihood maximization) the specific
   numeric model parameters that best fit the observations gathered in the
   training sample;
7. assess how well the model fits the data, each prognostic factor's
   statistical significance, in which direction each factor points, the

"shape" of each predictive relationship, and each factor's relative predictive potency—typically involving successive model refinements;

8. if the refined prognostic model statistically fitted to the training data achieves at least minimal adequacy, derive from it an explicit prognostic algorithm whose inputs (independent variables) are observations on the set of prognostic factors and whose output (dependent variable) is a prediction of the focal end point;

9. apply the prognostic algorithm to each patient in the training sample to obtain individually tailored predictions of the focal end point; and

10. assess the accuracy of the resulting tailored predictions.

Traditional prognostic research tends to focus on step seven, above. Executing steps eight, nine, and ten is only carried out to generate some measure of the factors' collective explanatory efficacy (e.g., R squared, their coefficient of determination). The point of the research is not to make any statements about any particular patient. It is to generate conclusions about the prognostic factors generalizable to some prespecified population of patients.

Research conclusions are statistical inferences about the target population. Inferences are drawn from careful analysis of sample observations. However, from a deductive perspective, the target population must be specified first. Then, both the sample of patients on which statistical inferences are based and the targeted individual patient must belong to that prespecified population.

More widely generalizable research conclusions (e.g., more-encompassing definitions of the target population) are typically judged as an indicator of higher-quality research.

These observations have three consequences.

1. Research conclusions based on isolated or otherwise limited samples (e.g., on patients drawn from a single institution) are frequently criticized as "biased", "unrepresentative", or "not population-based." They are suspected not to be representative of some more-comprehensive and, therefore, more-interesting overall patient population.

2. Research conclusions are presented as attributes of the prognostic factors rather than as attributes of individual patients. They are displayed in tables organized factor-by-factor, not patient-by-patient. They are descriptive statements about the factors themselves. They say nothing about individual patients.

   Thus, conclusions from a Cox (proportional hazards) regression analysis are typically tabled values of the estimated regression coefficients, their corresponding relative risks (hazard ratios), and their corresponding p values and calculated confidence intervals—a separate row in the table for each prognostic factor. Individually tailored survival curves, although easily producible from these tabled values, are rarely generated, graphed, or even mentioned.

   Conclusions from a logistic regression analysis are similarly presented as tabled values of the estimated regression coefficients, their corresponding odds ratios, and their corresponding p values and calculated confidence intervals. Again, individually tailored focal end point probabilities, although easily computable from these tabled values, are rarely produced, displayed, or even mentioned.

3. The subsequent operations required to move from step seven to step ten, above, are either omitted or not emphasized because the reason for executing them and their interpretation are not "general."

Empirical science is sometimes characterized as the search for relationships among empirical variables within some general context. Consistent with this view, steps one through seven, above, are all about the contemporary science of prognostic modeling. Steps eight, nine, and ten translate an evidence-based prognostic model into something useful to the artful practice of medicine. As an art, medicine is practiced patient-by-patient, not factor-by-factor.

It is most illuminating to note that making the translation interchanges the means-ends role of prognostic factors and individual patients.

While trying to establish predictive relationships between prognostic factors and focal states, events, and situations during steps one through seven, data obtained from individual patients are used to draw conclusions about prognostic factors. This is a factor-centered reasoning process. Conclusions are about the factors. Individual patient data serve as a means of (a basis for) drawing such conclusions. Individual patients are freely added to or removed from the training sample as a matter of analytical convenience—according to their role in contributing to appropriate conclusions about the factors. A patient who is not from the prespecified population or who possesses missing values on one or more prognostic factors is frequently deleted from the analysis.

While trying to draw a specific conclusion about an individual patient during steps eight, nine, and ten, prognostic factors provide the data source. This is a patient-centered reasoning process. Conclusions are about each separate patient. Conclusions are generated by executing an explicit prognostic algorithm applied, separately, to each patient. Particular factors are added to and removed from the algorithm as a matter of analytical convenience—according to their role in contributing to accurate predictions about individual patients. The very idea of completely ignoring (i.e., drawing no conclusion about) any patient because of missing data on one or more (but not all) prognostic factors is fundamentally antithetical to the goal of becoming patient-centered.

It seems fruitless to debate whether the prognostic factors or the individual patients constitute the "proper" or "more important" focus of medical research. It has just been demonstrated that a detailed consideration of each is necessary to draw evidence-based conclusions about the other.

On the other hand, it is probably useful to keep firmly in mind what is currently being viewed as a means toward achieving which goal in steps one through seven versus in steps eight, nine, and ten. They imply different directions of inference. Different directions of inference, in turn, often require different enabling procedures and different measures of success. All of these observations have important consequences that will be elaborated as the details of PCM are presented.

Note that the ten-step PCM does not begin with the specification of a target population. It begins with the identification of a targeted individual patient. We can think of it as the next patient freshly diagnosed with a particular cancer. For purposes of statistical inference, the relevant population is specified in steps one and two according to certain attributes of this next patient. The population includes all patients similar to this next patient— similar in terms of our practical ability to make an accurate prediction of the targeted patient's focal end point. It is by tailoring the subsequent analysis to each patient, separately, that the methodology becomes patient-centered.

Implementing PCM would require large amounts of thoroughly verified patient data and a currently nonexistent, institutionally shared infrastructure to maintain and update patient records over time. This will be discussed later.

The transition from a factor-centered to a patient-centered approach should be viewed as an important shift in methodology. The shift is to a different, though intimately interrelated research paradigm. Yet nothing is being discarded or replaced. Hence, the transition might best be characterized as a significantly reoriented paradigm enhancement, rather than as a fundamental paradigm shift.

These ten steps encapsulate the PCM approach to making tailored prognoses for individual patients. The most striking differences between what is being proposed here and the traditional prognostic paradigm lie both in the way the relevant patient population is initially specified and in the nature of the final conclusions. Traditional versions of the first seven steps generate general conclusions about the relative potency of various prognostic factors in some prespecified patient population of substantial professional interest. Selectively modifying the first seven steps, and then executing the last three steps, generate individually tailored patient predictions.

Various modifications will be made to all steps in the analytical procedure. These are designed to operationalize the patient-centered concept and to improve, thereby, individually tailored prognostic accuracy.

1.2 An Historical Trigger

In an article published in the *New England Journal of Medicine* in December 2006, titled The Limitations of Risk Factors as Prognostic Tools, Dr. James H. Ware commented, "Despite the strong association between [some] risk factor and [some] disease outcome, it does not follow that the risk factor provides a basis for an effective prediction rule for individual patients."

Dr. Ware's comment cut right to the core of the distinction between being factor-centered and becoming patient-centered. It suggested an improvement strategy. Could altering the fundamental goal of the methodology and modifying, accordingly, various operations, procedures, and techniques throughout the analysis improve individual predictive accuracy?

Dr. Ware reviewed an article by Whang and colleagues published in the same issue of the *New England Journal of Medicine*. Ten novel biomarkers were introduced as candidates for predicting both major cardiovascular events and death from any cause among 3,209 patients. Cox regression was the statistical technique used to assess these prognostic factors. After a stepwise (backward elimination) procedure, and after adjusting for conventional risk factors included as a base case in the multivariate analysis, Whang and colleagues identified five of these ten biomarkers as independently statistically significant. To measure the cumulative predictive contribution of the five significant biomarkers a weighted average biomarker score was constructed, using as weights the Cox regression coefficients estimated from the analysis.

Dr. Ware then concluded, "Despite this significant contribution to the [Cox] proportional hazards regression model, the proposed biomarker score adds little to the sensitivity and specificity of a prognostic test for death within five years. The usual measure of the performance of a prognostic test is the receiver-operating-characteristic [ROC] curve ... [and] the area under that curve [AUC]." By adding the five statistically significant novel biomarkers to a model that was based on conventional risk factors Whang and colleagues were able to boost their AUC by the equivalent of just two percentage points (from 0.795 to 0.816).

Dr. Ware's 2006 *New England Journal* article was the historical trigger for the development of PCM. Even when the factors added to a multivariate analysis are highly significant statistically, Dr. Ware pointed out that this fails to guarantee any substantial increase in individually tailored prognostic performance. Could a way be found to increase prognostic accuracy at the individual patient level beyond the typically modest (e.g., two-point) bump in AUC provided by simply adding novel prognostic factors to a standard list of conventional factors within the traditional, factor-centered research paradigm?

PCM was designed in direct response to Dr. Ware's challenge.

1.3 How PCM Differs from Traditional Prognostic Methodology

Although squarely rooted in traditional prognostic methodology, PCM possesses six differentiating characteristics.

  1. Altered Focus

    PCM focuses on individual patients rather than on selected prognostic factors. The analysis begins with a targeted individual patient rather than with an interesting patient population. A training sample is selected on the basis of that targeted patient's particular characteristics. The analysis then proceeds, separately, for separate training samples. The analysis ends with specific predictions about targeted patients rather than with general conclusions about the role and relative potency of prognostic factors in the interesting population.

    Beginning with a targeted individual patient has an important practical consequence. Imagine an Internet-based service center capable of making individually tailored prognoses for a number of different cancers. A patient enters descriptive information, such as demographic characteristics, family history, detailed diagnosis, current stage of the cancer's development, and so forth. The service center performs a tailored analysis on the spot. It returns a probabilistic prediction that the patient will or will not experience selected future outcomes and a probabilistic estimate of how long it will take for such outcomes to materialize. PCM would facilitate just such a service center.

    Since PCM's focus is on patients, not on prognostic factors, the ultimate purpose of any PCM analysis is neither to estimate nor to test statistical hypotheses concerning distributional parameters that characterize the impact of various prognostic factors in the population. Producing such estimates and performing such formal hypothesis tests do occur along the way. Nevertheless, these are only penultimate activities. They are the means to deriving separate conclusions about individual patients. The ultimate objective of PCM is to estimate, probabilistically, whether or not and when individual patients will experience specific outcomes. Formal hypothesis tests relate to which of two or more separate analytical procedures produce more accurate estimates and whether or not one such procedure is significantly superior to another in this respect.

    PCM's altered focus requires different measures of prognostic success. Novel success measures must be devised. After considering the traditional measures of factor success, such as significant p values and clinically important hazard ratios, specific measures of predictive accuracy at the individual patient level must be added. PCM's success is measured by ROC/AUC scores, rates of correct outcome prediction, probabilistic prediction errors, and appropriate predictive scale characteristics. Only ROC/AUC scores are familiar to most researchers.

All along the way, PCM relies heavily on traditional prognostic methodology. It uses a modified form of logistic regression analysis to predict the occurrence or nonoccurrence of medical events for a particular patient. It uses a modified form of Cox (proportional hazards) regression to generate individually tailored survival curves.

PCM extends traditional methodology. After drawing the usual factor-centered conclusions, it uses an explicit prognostic algorithm to make individually tailored, patient-centered predictions.

2. Selective Focus

PCM focuses exclusively on a particular end point. The focal end point is some salient patient outcome (i.e., state, event, or situation related to a targeted patient). Changing the focal end point always changes the detailed analyses performed and typically changes many analytical conclusions.

Because of its individual patient orientation, PCM does not seek to generate substantive medical conclusions generalizable either across patients or across focal end points. Its purpose is to make an accurate prediction of a focal end point for a targeted patient.

3. Selective Stratification

For many cancers, there exists a single prognostic factor or a single prognostic index constructed from more than one factor that is widely understood within the medical profession and regularly recorded for most patients. Primary tumor size or thickness is such a single factor. Stage of disease progression is such an index.

PCM selects from among such widely understood and regularly recorded factors and indexes the one that appears to possess the greatest univariate impact. Greatest impact means greatest ability to discriminate reliably among different patients in terms of disease progression—whether or not and how quickly the focal end point occurs.

The selected factor or index is then used to stratify the overall patient population. Separate strata contain distinct subpopulations of patients, where the strata differ significantly in terms of the incidence of and elapsed-time-to-reach the focal end point.

A training sample is drawn from the stratum (subpopulation) regarded as most similar to the targeted patient. Similarity refers to accuracy in predicting the focal end point. A prognostic model is trained on (fitted to data within) the similar-patient training sample to produce an explicit prognostic algorithm.

Selective stratification serves to homogenize patients within subpopulations. Simultaneously, it introduces heterogeneity across separate strata. This dual consequence of stratification is subsequently exploited by PCM. Statistical modeling is performed separately within homogenized subpopulations. This tends to improve the fit of prognostic models (e.g., logistic regression and Cox regression) to training data. Missing observations are handled separately across heterogeneous strata. This renders the likely consequence of a missing patient observation related to some particular prognostic factor easier to estimate.

If no suitable factor or index exists for a given cancer, the patient population is not stratified. When performed, the differentiating consequences of stratification are verified. The differential incidence of and elapsed-time-to-reach the focal end point across subpopulations are both tested statistically (e.g., via Kaplan-Meier analysis).

Selective stratification is one of the principal devices by which PCM improves individually tailored prognostic accuracy.

4. SPSA Conversion

The Scale Partitioning and Spacing Algorithm (SPSA) is another device to improve prognostic accuracy. Scale partitioning means that the set of possible raw measurement values of a prognostic factor is subdivided into two or more distinct subscales. Scale partitioning is optimized so as to produce the most sensitive and specific prediction of the focal end point. Spacing means ascertaining the apparent "distances" separating partitioned subscales that reveal the "shape" of the univariate relationship linking a prognostic factor to the focal end point. The result is a Univariate Impact-Reflecting Index (UIRI). The raw measurement scale of most prognostic factors is uniformly converted by SPSA into a corresponding UIRI.

A UIRI indicates the direction, shape and magnitude of whatever univariate relationship the training data suggest may exist between each prognostic factor and the focal end point. Direction of impact indicates how more or less of the factor relates to more or less of its impact on the focal end point. Shape of relationship indicates whether the factor's impact is exerted at a constant, accelerating, or decelerating rate at different factor levels. Magnitude of impact indicates the prognostic factor's apparent clinical importance relative to the focal end point.

A UIRI is depicted both graphically and algebraically. Its algebraic form is normally incorporated into the prognostic model (explicit algorithm) produced by PCM for a training sample. Its graphical depiction is for human consumption.

SPSA is a useful tool to the extent that a prognostic factor's impact on some focal end point is genuine, though incompletely understood.

A UIRI indicates correlation in the training data. It may or may not also indicate a causal connection linking the prognostic factor to the focal end point. Fortunately, since prediction is the goal of PCM, mere correlation, when genuine, can still be useful, as long as it is systematic. The underlying biology need not be understood in detail.

Genuine means that the apparent linkage relationship is more than a statistical artifact resulting from overfitting a prognostic model to inadequate training data. Large training samples are required to distinguish genuine relationships (even if only correlational) from spurious correlations. Only large samples can support split-sample reliability testing, whereby the predictive improvements seemingly achieved in a training sample can be shown to carry over to a validation sample.

On the other hand, if the detailed biological mechanisms mediating a factor's impact were well-understood, raw data conversion via SPSA would not be helpful. It would not be performed. Yet detailed knowledge of the underlying pathways and connections linking commonly used prognostic factors to popular focal end points is, today, largely nonexistent. Even the shape, as opposed to just the direction, of many such linkage relationships remains poorly understood.

PCM, therefore, converts almost all prognostic factor data into corresponding UIRI scores. This does not improve the univariate predictive accuracy of dichotomous prognostic factors, such as whether or not a primary tumor has become ulcerated. Such factors possess a directional relationship, but without any distinctive shape. In contrast, the predictive accuracy of genuinely quantitative prognostic factors, such as tumor size and mitotic rate, is sometimes improved substantially. Quantitative factors can display quite distinctive and predictively useful shapes.

5. Dealing with Missing Observations

A training sample may contain missing observations on one or more prognostic factors. If not too many observations were missing and if the goal of the analysis were factor-centered, it would be tempting simply to delete patients with missing observations from the analysis.

Becoming patient-centered, however, precludes such a strategy. The goal is to make a prognosis, even if imprecise, for all patients. SPSA includes detailed procedures to estimate likely end point values for missing observations of all prognostic factors. The efficacy of these procedures is considerably enhanced by selective stratification of the patient population.

SPSA's special handling of missing observations is another device that improves individually tailored prognostic accuracy.

6. Incorporating Additional Factors

The progress of medical science will continue to produce new prognostic factors for various cancers. Incorporating new factors into the analysis via stratification, SPSA, and its special handling of missing observations seems especially helpful. The addition of substantial biological information analyzed in this manner improves prognostic accuracy even further.

It will later be shown that, when additional factors are incorporated into the prognostic analysis via PCM using all of these devices together, AUC increases in the range of ten to fifteen points can be achieved.

Such increases were achieved in the PCM analysis of 1,222 melanoma patients from the United States and in a separate PCM analysis of 1,225 breast cancer patients from Finland. In the case of the Finnish patients, a final AUC value of 0.900 was achieved.

These results compare quite favorably with the two-point bump, ending up with a final AUC value of 0.816, discussed by Dr. Ware. He was reporting what Whang and colleagues were able to accomplish by adding five new statistically significant biomarkers to a prognostic analysis of cardiovascular events performed with traditional methodology.

2.0 RECONSTRUCTING CURRENT PROGNOSTIC METHODOLOGY

Following Dr. Ware's lead, we begin by distinguishing between:

1. traditional or conventional prognostic risk factors widely understood at a particular moment in history and utilized to make predictions about a particular cancer; and
2. additional factors subsequently identified by ongoing medical research in that same field.

We shall modify currently employed analytical procedures in a manner consistent with our enhanced, patient-centered research paradigm (PCM). This is what we mean by reconstructing current prognostic methodology.

Current prognostic methodology will first be applied to the conventional risk factors. This will establish a base case for all subsequent comparisons.

The modified procedures will then be applied to exactly the same observational data. Can we improve prognostic accuracy for an individual patient simply by systematically changing the way we analyze conventional and traditional factors? If so, our second task will be to apply the procedural modifications to the analysis of additional prognostic factors as they are discovered through ongoing medical research.

Does this provide still further improvements? If so, our third task will be to calibrate the relative improvement in prognostic accuracy realizable, first, just by moving from a factor-centered to a patient-centered methodology and then, by adding new prognostic factors analyzed via PCM. To determine which of these procedural modifications and which new prognostic factors are actually contributing to the improvement, as well as their interactions, their predictive efficacy relative to one another will be systematically compared.

A sequence of operations, procedures, and techniques—selectively modified to achieve a patient-centered orientation—is presented in the following subsections.

2.1 Selecting a Focal End Point

Salient events in the progression of melanoma and breast cancer include:

1. initial diagnosis;
2. undergoing a specified treatment;
3. local metastasis of the primary tumor;
4. regional metastasis to a nearby lymphatic basin;
5. distant metastasis to a location far removed from the primary tumor; and
6. death of the patient, possibly due to the cancer itself.

Prognosis typically spans the time interval between either a patient's initial diagnosis or some specified treatment and one of these subsequent events. Whatever is selected as the outcome of interest is defined as the focal end point. Predicting the occurrence of the selected event then becomes the focus of the prognostic effort.

Predictions of events can be stated in any of several ways.

1. When the focal event is defined as the outcome of some test procedure with either a positive or a negative result, the prediction is dichotomous. Thus, a sentinel lymph node biopsy performed on either a melanoma or a breast cancer patient may be either positive, indicating that the cancer has already penetrated the lymphatic system, or negative, providing no evidence of such penetration to date. A positive biopsy is typically designated the focal event. A negative biopsy is typically designated the alternative or complementary event.

2. When the focal event is defined as local, regional, or distant metastasis within a specified interval of time following initial diagnosis, the prediction is also dichotomous. A patient may either survive for five years or ten years without experiencing such an event or not survive that long event-free. Experiencing the event within the specified interval is typically designated the focal event. Surviving event-free beyond the specified interval is typically designated the alternative or complementary event.

3. When the length of the time interval following initial diagnosis required for a focal event to occur is being predicted, the prediction is not dichotomous. It is a continuous, nonnegative magnitude.

4. When an event-free survival time following either initial diagnosis or some specified treatment is being predicted, the prediction is also not dichotomous. It, too, is a continuous, nonnegative magnitude.

How a prediction is stated determines what type of prognostic analysis may be performed. Logistic regression is a popular and statistically powerful analysis technique for making dichotomous (one of two mutually exclusive) predictions. Kaplan-Meier analysis and Cox (proportional hazards) regression are frequently the techniques of choice for predicting the likely duration of survival times. These techniques will be employed and illustrated as the discussion proceeds.

Prognosis always begins with the selection of a focal event. If more than one focal event is to be predicted, at least partially and sometimes completely separate analyses may be required—a separate analysis to support the prediction of each separate focal event. This can occur because of differences in the nature of the desired prediction (e.g., a dichotomous event versus the magnitude of some elapsed time interval). It can also occur because the same prognostic factors may be related quite differently to different focal events (e.g., the same genes may play different roles in mediating local, regional, and distant metastasis).

We claim that the utility of PCM is not restricted to any single cancer (or, for that matter, only to cancer). To demonstrate this, we have applied the same methodology to two different cancers. It has been applied both to a sample of 1,222 melanoma patients and to a distinct and completely unrelated sample of 1,225 invasive breast cancer patients.

Appropriate comparisons between these two applications requires judicious selection of a common focal event. Disease-specific death within five years following initial diagnosis was chosen as the common focal event. This choice was motivated by the following considerations.

1. Consistent with Dr. Ware's comments, we adopted ROC/AUC analysis as an appropriate way to judge the performance of an individually tailored prognostic test.

2. This suggested, although it did not require defining the focal event in dichotomous terms. We adopted logistic regression rather than Cox regression as the best available analytical technique for making

dichotomous predictions.
3. Overall death is a popular end point in many prognostic studies. Disease-specific death is of decidedly greater interest both to cancer patients and to their doctors. It is perhaps the single most salient end point one might choose.
4. In addition, our research has shown consistently better prognostic results for disease-specific death and disease-specific survival (DSS) than for overall death and overall survival (OS).
5. It was possible to determine cause of death in both our sample of 1,222 melanoma patients and our sample of 1,225 breast cancer patients.
6. Five-year and ten-year outcomes are popular dichotomous choices in prognostic studies. The duration of patient follow-up in both of our samples (averaging between five and ten years) was adequate to support the prediction of five-year, but not ten-year disease-specific death.
7. Historical data on five-year, but not ten-year disease-specific survival drawn from a sample containing more than ten thousand fairly recent melanoma patients all over the world were available to us. These data were stratified according to each patient's disease stage at the time of initial diagnosis. Such results provided a convenient basis of comparison for our sample of 1,222 melanoma patients.
8. No compelling arguments supported a different feasible choice.

2.2 Selecting Individually Tailored Measures to Calibrate Prognostic Accuracy

As just indicated, choosing a dichotomous focal event suggested using logistic regression as our principal analytical tool. The usual outputs of a logistic regression analysis are easily modifiable to produce a tailored prediction for each patient in a sample so analyzed.

Excluding both patients who die within five years of something else unrelated to their cancer and patients who are followed up for no more than five years, a patient either dies of metastatic cancer within five years of diagnosis, or that patient survives for more than five years. Patients were excluded from both our melanoma and our breast cancer samples according to these two restrictions. In each case, excluded patients accounted for between 5 and 10 percent of those patients who otherwise qualified for inclusion.

The mathematical model underlying logistic regression assumes that the natural logarithm of the betting odds associated with a dichotomous focal event, such as death from metastatic cancer within five years after diagnosis, is the following linear function of some set of K prognostic factors:

$$Y = B0 + (B1)(X1) + (B2)(X2) + \ldots + (BK)(XK), \text{ where}$$

Y, the single dependent variable, is the natural logarithm of the ratio of the probability of occurrence of the focal event (disease-specific death within five years) to the complementary probability that the event will not occur (five-year disease-specific survival);

X1, X2, ... , XK are the K prognostic factor(s) serving as independent variables;

B0 is the "intercept" or constant-value-added regression coefficient;

B1, B2, ... , BK are the K logistic regression coefficient(s) associated, respectively, with each of the K independent variable(s); and the values of all K independent variables and of all K + 1 logistic regression coefficients are positive or negative real numbers or zero.

Once a logistic regression analysis has been performed, revised, and deemed at least minimally adequate, an estimated probability of occurrence of the focal event may be assigned to each separate patient according to the following prognostic algorithm:

EXP[B0 + (B1)(X1) + (B2)(X2) + ... + (BK)(XK)]/{1 + EXP[B0 + (B1)(X1) + (B2)(X2) + ... + (BK)(XK)]}, where

EXP means to exponentiate the immediately following bracketed expression relative to the natural logarithm base;

B0, B1, ... , BK are the numeric values of the regression coefficients estimated by the logistic analysis; and

X1, X2, ... , XK are the numerically coded values of that patient's prognostic factors.

As with any statistical analysis, there is the problem of how to deal with missing or inadmissible observations. The two previously described restrictions eliminated missing data on the dependent variable. Section 2.7 describes how we dealt with this problem with respect to missing observations on all independent variables (prognostic factors) in both of our samples.

Using the above algorithm we can make an individually tailored prediction of the focal event for every patient in the sample. The prediction is a probability that each patient experiences the focal event (disease-specific death within five years of diagnosis). These individually tailored probabilities constitute our principal patient-centered prognostic measure. The algorithm assigns such a probability to any patient, including patients not included in the logistic regression analysis, as a function of that patient's numeric values of the K prognostic factors.

Had we defined our focal event in terms of the time interval between diagnosis and disease-specific death, analogous individually tailored probabilities could have been generated by performing a Cox regression analysis on the same K prognostic factors.

The proportional hazards model underlying Cox regression assumes that the population from which the sample was obtained possesses a baseline hazard function of this elapsed time interval. Each patient's individual hazard function is assumed to be directly proportional to the shared baseline hazard function. Each patient possesses a separate proportionality factor that is independent of the elapsed time interval. It is calculated by exponentiating the following homogeneous linear function of the K prognostic factors:

Y = EXP[(B1)(X1) + (B2)(X2) + ... + (BK)(XK)], where

Y is a given patient's proportionality factor which is to be multiplied by the shared baseline hazard function to obtain that patient's individual hazard function; and where EXP and the B, X, and K values are defined as in logistic regression, except that B1 through BK are now Cox regression coefficients.

Associated with the baseline hazard function is a baseline survival function of the same elapsed time interval. It, too, is shared by all patients in the population. Cox regression analysis can be programmed to produce both baseline functions. The individually tailored prognostic algorithm generated from Cox regression then uses each patient's proportionality factor to exponentiate the baseline survival function. Applying this algorithm to a particular patient's prognostic factors and evaluating the resulting function at a particular elapsed time interval (five years) gives an individually tailored (five-year) survival probability. Conceptually, this is the complement of the focal event probability generated by logistic regression from the same prognostic factors.

Next, we need measures of predictive accuracy. We have chosen four.

1. Following Dr. Ware's suggestion, the individually tailored probabilities assigned by the prognostic algorithm to any set of patients may be submitted to a traditional ROC/AUC analysis. A numeric AUC value between 0.0 and 1.0 may be estimated from such a sample of probabilities. The larger the estimated AUC value, the better that prognostic algorithm may be judged as discriminating among patients in the sample in terms of whether or not each one experiences the focal event. An AUC value of 1.0 indicates perfect discrimination.

2. Another way to judge accuracy may be derived from the same set of individually tailored probabilities. First, rank-order them from largest to smallest. Then, test each cut point between adjacent probabilities in the rank order as a possible dichotomous discriminator. Tentatively, predict that all patients whose probabilities exceed a given cut point experience the focal event, while all patients with lower probabilities do not. Count the number of correct predictions for that cut point. Choose the cut point that offers the highest correct count. Define this count as the maximum possible number (or percentage) of correct predictions. An AUC value of 1.0 implies a 100 percent correct prediction rate, and vice versa.

3. Absolute probabilistic error provides another measure. This is the absolute value of the difference between each patient's probability of experiencing the focal event and what actually occurs. Actual occurrence is coded as 1.0. Actual nonoccurrence is coded as 0.0. The absolute difference is useful in comparing the accuracy of two or more alternative methods of generating tailored individual probabilities (i.e., via two or more alternative prognostic algorithms). The statistical power of matched sample analysis can then be exploited to conclude which generation method provides more accurate probabilities.

4. Because individually tailored focal event probabilities are not all that familiar in traditional prognostic research methodology it is useful to ascertain their scale characteristics. Most conveniently, logistic regression guarantees that they are accurate on the average. The mean probability assigned by logistic regression to a sample of patients is numerically equal to the incidence (relative frequency) of the focal event in that sample. Less conveniently, Cox regression does not guarantee the same average accuracy. Yet what about individually tailored probabilities at the lower and upper extremes of the probability scale? Even when correct on the average, does predictive accuracy deteriorate in the case of small and large probabilities? By partitioning the probability scale (e.g., into quartiles), similar comparisons may be repeated between mean probabilities and actual incidences throughout the entire scale.

2.3   Establishing a Base Case for Assessing Accuracy Improvements

For a number of years the American Joint Committee on Cancer (AJCC) has been focusing on certain prognostic factors useful in predicting the progress of both melanoma and breast cancer. For melanoma, prior to 2009, these included:

1. age of patient at the time of initial diagnosis (whole number of years
   as of most recent birthday—risk increases with age);
2. sex of patient (male or female—male higher risk);
3. anatomical location of primary tumor (axial, if on head, neck, or
   trunk; peripheral, if on arms or legs—axial higher risk);
4. thickness of primary tumor (Breslow depth in millimeters—risk
   increases with thickness);
5. Clark level of tumor invasion (I, II, III, IV, or V—risk increases
   with Clark level); and
6. ulceration of primary tumor (present or absent—ulcerated tumors higher
   risk).

Higher risk in terms of experiencing disease-specific death means either a
higher likelihood of dying from metastatic cancer within five years of initial
diagnosis or a shorter anticipated time interval until experiencing that focal
event.

In 2009, the AJCC announced the substitution of mitotic rate for Clark level if
the mitotic rate observed within the primary tumor is ascertainable at the time
of initial diagnosis. Mitotic rate is a nonnegative count per hpf (high-powered
field). Mitotic rate, when ascertainable, was also substituted for Clark level
in the revised AJCC melanoma staging classification for 2010 and beyond. Risk
increases with mitotic rate. [Technical note: a high-powered field (hpf) in our
mitotic rate data was interpreted as one square millimeter.]

We adopted these revised AJCC six prognostic factors as the base case against
which to assess accuracy improvements in our sample of 1,222 melanoma patients.
It will be designated the factor-centered base case. We also adopted the
revised AJCC melanoma staging classification as an indicator of each patient's
level of risk at the time of initial diagnosis. Data on all six traditional
factors and initial stage were available for melanoma patients.

To achieve comparability, we began with the following six prognostic factors
available in the data set describing our sample of 1,225 invasive breast cancer
patients as their factor-centered base case:

1. age of patient at the time of initial diagnosis (whole number of years
   as of most recent birthday—risk increases with age);
2. sex of patient (male or female—but no males in the sample);
3. anatomical location of primary tumor within breast (central, lateral,
   medial, or diffuse—diffuse higher risk);
4. size of primary tumor along its longest dimension (in millimeters—
   risk increases with tumor size);
5. mitotic count of primary tumor (per hpf—risk increases with mitotic
   count); and
6. ulceration of primary tumor (present or absent—ulcerated tumors higher
   risk).

All 1,225 breast cancer patients were female. Consequently, sex of patient
could not be used as a discriminating prognostic factor.

AJCC staging classification data were not recorded in our data set describing
breast cancer patients. Fortunately, observations on each patient's T, N, and M
scales were. Since T, N, and M values are the principal ingredients used to
construct AJCC stage (a composite index), we applied the published 2010 AJCC
staging classification scheme to each patient's T, N, and M observations. This
generated an initial stage for most (approximately 96 percent) of our breast
cancer patients.

2.4 Stratifying Patients According to Risk of Experiencing the Focal Event

Recall that our proposed patient-centered methodology begins:

1. not with an interesting, prespecified population to which conclusions about the prognostic factors will be generalized, based on a carefully selected sample of patient data (this is the factor-centered approach);
2. but instead, with a particular patient whose specified focal event is to be predicted on the basis of carefully selected prognostic factors.

To begin with a particular patient means to define the population relevant from the standpoint of statistical inference in terms of that targeted patient. This is the reverse of the usual sequence. It also reinterprets the fundamental concept of representativeness.

In a patient-centered context, it is the population of patients selected as similar to the targeted individual patient that either succeeds or fails to succeed in being prognostically useful. To be useful, an appropriate segment or stratum of the totality of all patients must first be identified as similar enough to the targeted patient so that whatever happens to patients in that segment or stratum can reasonably be expected, also, to happen to the targeted patient. Data relevant to making the focal prediction must then be gathered on a sample of patients drawn strictly from that similar segment or stratum.

It is not necessarily virtuous in a patient-centered context for a sample to be total-population-based. Virtue now lies in being similar-segment-based. Of course, if a total population is homogeneous in all important respects, being similar-segment-based means the same thing as being total-population-based. There are no usefully distinguishable segments. Then, but only then is being total-population-based still a virtue.

To be virtuous, a sample must still be representative of and (at least treatable as if) drawn at random from this similar segment or stratum. Our patient-centered approach does not relax that requirement.

Seeking to identify a similar segment or stratum of a population for a targeted individual patient is hardly a new concept. Political pollsters, when trying to predict the outcome of an important election, and market researchers, when trying to predict customer response to various sales and marketing tactics, long ago discovered a frequently effective "divide and conquer" strategy. Pollsters call it stratified sampling. Marketers call it market segmentation.

The basic idea is this.

1. Start by asking if the total population is homogeneous or heterogeneous.
2. Homogeneity here refers to similarities in the prognostic connections linking certain observable characteristics of members of the total population (voters or customers or patients) to interesting outcomes (votes cast or purchases made or the occurrence of focal events).
3. If the total population is everywhere homogeneous in this respect, forget the "divide and conquer" strategy. It will not help.
4. Alternatively, if the total population, though heterogeneous as a whole, possesses identifiable pockets of homogeneity, stratify or segment accordingly and exploit the within-segment homogeneity in making selective predictions.
5. Political pollsters learned that conducting a stratified random sample of separately heterogeneous voting precincts, with each one internally

homogeneous in terms of typical voting patterns, is far more
cost-effective than conducting a simple random sample of an entire
heterogeneous voting population.

6. Marketers learned that sending separately tailored promotional messages
to identifiably different segments of the total market populated by
customers with different incomes, needs, and worldviews is frequently
more effective than sending the same, "one shoe fits all" promotional
message to everybody.

By analogy, we start by asking if the total patient population for some cancer
is homogeneous or heterogeneous. Such populations appear to be heterogeneous in
many prognostic respects, but with identifiable pockets of homogeneity.

The salient end points we typically try to predict for both melanoma and breast
cancer patients include relapse or recurrence, distant metastasis, and death.
These events occur at successive stages of cancer progression. Consequently,
stratifying or segmenting any given patient population in terms of successive
stages of disease progression might well produce analytically exploitable
pockets of homogeneity.

These two observations suggest the following question. Can we first stratify
cancer patients according to their risk level (i.e., stage of disease
progression) at diagnosis and then separately perform all subsequent analytical
procedures? This means executing all analyses separately by risk category and
then merging separately and independently calculated results at the end.

In particular, it suggests using the AJCC staging classification for both
melanoma and breast cancer patients not as just another prognostic factor
(independent variable) in a multivariate statistical analysis. Instead, it
suggests using each as a stratifying factor that permits separate and
independent multivariate statistical analyses to be performed on all the other
admissible prognostic factors.

Whether or not and the extent to which any total population of cancer patients
is heterogeneous as a whole, but with pockets of exploitable homogeneity is an
empirical question. We do not just assume it. We try out various segmentation
principles and stratification criteria and check for predictive improvement.

It will be shown later that AJCC stage at diagnosis provides the highest-impact
basis for stratification in both our sample of 1,222 melanoma patients and our
sample of 1,225 breast cancer patients. It is superior to all of the other
well-understood and widely available traditional or conventional prognostic
factors in each case. More importantly, stratifying the analysis by AJCC stage
improves predictive accuracy in both cancers.

2.5 Admissibility Requirements for Traditional and Nontraditional Factors

Virtually any attribute of a patient or aspect of that patient's life situation
can serve as a candidate prognostic factor. However, not all candidates are
admissible. In order for a candidate attribute or aspect to qualify as an
admissible prognostic factor in our patient-centered methodology:

1. it must be recorded on a raw measurement scale containing at least two
distinguishable, numerically coded values—otherwise, it cannot serve
to discriminate among patients in terms of the focal event;
2. its raw measurement values (if the scale possesses three or more) must
indicate increasing or decreasing degrees of whatever attribute or

aspect is being measured—otherwise, it cannot be said to constitute at least an ordinal measure of that raw attribute or aspect;

3. it must be systematically related (either causally or correlationally) to the focal event—otherwise, it cannot be said to have any relevant prognostic impact;

4. where the systematic relationship must be monotonic throughout the entire scale of values—otherwise, the impact of the prognostic factor on the focal event cannot be said to be uniformly directional (how to verify uniform directionality will be discussed in section 2.6);

5. where the uniformly directional nature of the relationship must be reasonably well-established (e.g., in the relevant scientific literature) in advance of any patient-centered analysis—otherwise, the prognostic methodology cannot be characterized as plausibly predictive (as opposed to just exploratory); and

6. it must be available as raw data in a training sample of similar patients, and at least two distinct scale values must be assigned to patients in that sample—otherwise, it cannot be used to estimate statistically the parameters of a prognostic algorithm applicable to any individual patient, including the targeted patient.

These admissibility requirements apply to all traditional or conventional prognostic factors comprising the factor-centered base case. They apply equally to all nontraditional (perhaps newly discovered) prognostic factors that are subsequently added to the analysis.

Requiring candidate prognostic factors to possess a pre-established (in the literature) direction of impact on the focal event provides an important methodological protection. The protection is against statistical overfitting of the prognostic algorithm generated by the analysis to the training data contained in the sample of similar patients. Fitted relationships are based only on factors with a respectable, pre-existing track record. Hence, they are less likely to capitalize on the chance associations that frequently arise in small and medium-sized training samples.

A second line of defense against statistical overfitting is provided by the partitioning procedure described in section 2.6. Any candidate prognostic factor that fails to demonstrate, uniformly, the previously established directionality among separate partitions—each containing at least a minimum admissible partition size (i.e., count of patients in the subsample associated with that partition)—is deemed inadmissible and purged from the analysis.

Increasing the size of the training sample can then be counted on to improve genuine predictive accuracy. It does not just increase the opportunity to detect more random associations. We shall return to this theme in section 5, where final conclusions are drawn and recommendations are offered.

2.6 Partitioning Each Factor Scale to Optimize Univariate Discriminability

Discrimination is the principal benefit provided by any prognostic factor. Its role in the analysis is to indicate whether, when, and in what ways individual patients will experience a focal event. Univariate discriminability refers to the ability of any single factor to accomplish this, acting by itself and not in some multivariate concert with other factors.

The raw measurement scale of each admissible factor for which data are available in the training sample is separately processed by the Scale Partitioning and Spacing algorithm (SPSA) in the following manner.

1. If the desired prediction has not already been expressed in dichotomous form, a convenient dichotomous version of the prediction is constructed for partitioning purposes. For example, if it is expressed in terms of a continuous time interval until a focal event occurs, some standard time interval, such as five or ten years, may be used.
2. The training sample is initially divided into two subsamples: a focal subsample, containing those patients who actually experienced the focal event (disease-specific death within five years of diagnosis), and a complementary subsample, containing those who experienced the complementary event (survival for more than five years). Each subsample must contain at least one patient.
3. A Mann-Whitney test is performed on the two subsamples in terms of the factor's raw measurement values. This provides an initial admissibility check on the factor's proper directionality. If higher levels of the prognostic factor are associated, historically, with a higher risk of experiencing the focal event, the focal subsample should possess systematically higher raw measurement values than the complementary subsample.
4. Minimal admissibility is achieved as long as the factor does not point in the historically wrong direction. When achieved, historical admissibility is thereby verified for the current training sample.
5. The admissibility criterion can be strengthened by requiring some minimally acceptable value of the Mann-Whitney test's directional (one-tail) p value. When verified, it is the factor's scale of numerically coded raw measurement values that will be partitioned into ordered subscales and "spaced" by SPSA.
6. If the raw measurement scale contains only two values, or if only two distinct scale values are assigned to patients in the training sample, there is only one possible way to partition an historically admissible scale. Further verification of its proper direction of impact is now sought by imposing four additional, logically equivalent requirements.

   a. Assuming that the higher raw measurement value indicates higher risk, define the factor's impact (discrimination) sensitivity as the proportion of those patients in the focal subsample who received the higher-risk raw measurement value.
   b. Assuming that the lower raw measurement value indicates lower risk, define the factor's impact (discrimination) specificity as the proportion of those patients in the complementary subsample who received the lower-risk raw measurement value.
   c. The factor's impact sensitivity (when a true positive indication occurred) must exceed the proportion of patients in the complementary subsample who received the higher-risk raw measurement value (when a false positive indication occurred).
   d. The factor's impact specificity (when a true negative indication occurred) must exceed the proportion of patients in the focal subsample who received the lower-risk raw measurement value (when a false negative indication occurred).
   e. The proportion of those patients receiving the higher-risk (true positive) raw measurement value who actually experienced the focal event must exceed the proportion of those patients receiving the lower-risk (false negative) raw measurement value who actually experienced the focal event.
   f. The proportion of those patients receiving the lower-risk (true negative) raw measurement value who actually experienced the complementary event must exceed the proportion of those patients receiving the higher-risk (false positive) raw measurement value who actually experienced the complementary event.

If not further verified in this manner, the prognostic factor is inadmissible. It either points in no direction or it points in the wrong direction.

7. When proper directionality is so verified and when each of the two raw measurement values is assigned to a large enough subsample of patients, no further steps need be executed. These two values constitute the optimally partitioned scale for this prognostic factor. Each partition contains exactly one of the two raw measurement values. Proceed to "spacing" the two partitions by assigning Univariate Impact-Reflecting Index (UIRI) values. Otherwise, subsequent steps are required to partition the factor's at-least-three-valued raw measurement scale.

8. All possible cut points within the training sample of rank-ordered raw measurement values must be checked to further verify admissibility. If the factor's raw measurement scale contains N distinct values, there are N - 1 potential cut points separating adjacent pairs of values in the rank order.

9. An admissible cut point is one that both subdivides the training sample into two subsamples of patients—each containing at least a minimum admissible partition size—and preserves the historically determined direction of impact in the above four (logically equivalent) senses.

10. Every cut point defines a conceptual two-by-two cross-tabulated frequency table.

    a. The first row of such a conceptual table contains patients whose raw measurement value falls below the cut point.
    b. The second row contains patients with values at or above the cut point.
    c. The first column of such a conceptual table contains patients in the complementary subsample.
    d. The second column contains patients in the focal subsample.

The admissibility of any cut point can then be determined by constructing its conceptual two-by-two cross-tabulated frequency table and applying any of the same four (logically equivalent) requirements.

11. Assuming there exists at least one admissible cut point, the optimal cut point is the one among them that maximizes the mean of the impact sensitivity and impact specificity that it determines.

12. If the context of the analysis is such that achieving either impact sensitivity or impact specificity is deemed more important than the other, an appropriately weighted mean is maximized instead.

13. In either case, if the maximum is not unique, choose the cut point from the admissible set with the largest (weighted) mean sensitivity and specificity whose minimum-sized partition is largest.

14. In the absence of any admissible cut points, there is no optimum cut point, the factor's raw measurement scale is not partitioned, and the factor is declared inadmissible.

15. The raw measurement scale is actually partitioned into two subscales by the optimal cut point, assuming one is successfully identified. There is a lower subscale and a higher subscale. The total sample of patients is partitioned into corresponding lower and higher subsamples.

16. The preceding steps are then repeated, first for each lower subscale and its corresponding lower subsample, and then for each higher subscale and its corresponding higher subsample.

17. Successive repetitions continue, as long as optimum cut points, optimum sub-cut points, optimum sub-sub-cut points, and so forth, continue to be identified.

18. At each step in the process where the repeated procedure generates either a lower or a higher subscale or both and when either or both subscales are subsequently partitioned, additional directionality

checks are also required across partitionings. Failure to pass such an additional check serves to invalidate the corresponding subsequent partitioning, but it does not invalidate any successful prior partitionings.

A candidate prognostic factor may be eliminated as inadmissible because it points in no direction or because it points in the historically wrong direction or because it fails to generate at least two raw measurement scale partitions, each one of sufficiently large corresponding subsample size.

The maximum number of scale partitions that can be produced by this SPSA algorithm is the number of distinct raw measurement values assigned to patients in a training sample. The maximum number is only achieved when each distinct raw value occupies a separate partition (subscale). In practice, however, our experience suggests that only a few common prognostic factors for predicting cancer produce more than five separate impact-reflecting scale partitions. It is true that many such factors possess more than five values in their raw measurement scales (e.g., scales measuring tumor size in millimeters), but their effective discriminating power generally supports no more than five when SPSA is actually executed with a reasonably large minimum partition size.

2.7 Assigning Impact-Reflecting Index Values to Partitioned Factor Subscales

Univariate Impact-Reflecting Index (UIRI) values are designed to produce an appropriate "spacing" among optimally partitioned subscales of a prognostic factor's raw measurement scale. UIRI values are coded either as uniformly nonnegative numbers (the usual case) or as uniformly nonpositive numbers. The numbers are calculated to reflect the relative magnitudes of impact (possibly causal, possibly correlational) linking each factor's ordered sequence of partitioned subscales to the focal event. Even when neither fully understood nor explained in detail, such impacts are presumed actually to exist.

Section 2.6 generates optimal cut points that guarantee the partitioning of each admissible prognostic factor scale into two or more subscales. Each subscale is associated with a subsample containing at least a minimum number of patients. Successive subscales are guaranteed to be uniformly directional in their impact on the focal event. That is, falling into one of the two or more ordered subscales indicates monotonically greater (or lesser) probability that the focal event will occur or monotonically shorter (or longer) time intervals until the focal event occurs or monotonically shorter (or longer) survival times.

Whereas section 2.6 guarantees the proper ordering of factor impacts, this subsection attempts to "space," quantitatively, successive subscales according to their relative magnitudes of impact. An appropriate "spacing" of a factor's impact identifies the general "shape" of its relationship to the focal event.

UIRI values are constructed for logistic regression by means of zero-one dummy variables. Dummy variables are assigned to the ordered sequence of optimally partitioned subscales produced in section 2.6. The dummy variables are constructed to identify in which partitioned subsample each patient belongs. When the logistic regression coefficients estimated for these dummy variables are transformed via the prediction algorithm presented in section 2.2 into individual patient probabilities of experiencing the focal event, these probabilities become UIRI values. Analogous UIRI values will shortly be constructed via the same dummy-variable technique for Cox regression.

Numerically equivalent UIRI values may sometimes be obtained in a much simpler manner. In the context of logistic regression, the principal predictive measure is the probability that each individual patient will experience the focal event. A reasonable estimate of the probability that any randomly selected patient whose raw prognostic factor value falls into a particular subscale will experience the focal event is, therefore, the proportion of such patients in the corresponding training subsample who actually do experience it.

Conveniently, UIRI values produced by dummy-variable logistic regression are numerically equivalent to observed subsample relative frequencies. If one patient's raw factor value falls within a factor subscale whose associated relative frequency is some number of percentage units greater than some other patient's associated relative frequency, a proportionately larger impact on the probability of occurrence of the focal event is inferred.

We account for missing or unavailable observations in a uniform manner. All such observations on any prognostic factor are collected in a single, additional subscale. All patients possessing these missing observations are collected into a corresponding additional training subsample. Just as with nonmissing observations, the missing subscale must be of at least the minimum partition size. Then, a reasonable estimate of the probability that any randomly selected patient whose raw prognostic factor value falls within the missing subscale will experience the focal event is the proportion of such patients in the corresponding training subsample who actually do experience it.

Adding a third or any additional subscale and corresponding training subsample to account for missing observations in this uniform manner assumes that no systematically different reasons for being missing are known. It is analogous to assuming that no systematically different reasons are known for producing censored observations in Kaplan-Meier analysis and Cox regression analysis.

Also, too sparsely populated a missing observation subsample (and subscale) is combined in a nonbiasing manner with a nonmissing subsample (and subscale) contiguous in terms of observed focal event relative frequency.

The need for a minimum subscale partition size (i.e., associated subsample size) should now be apparent. Cut points that partition a raw measurement scale into subscales associated with too small subsamples of patients should be avoided. Otherwise, relative frequencies used to calculate impact-reflecting index values will provide statistically unstable spacing (magnitude) estimates.

Practical application of the patient-centered methodology contemplates training samples containing at least thousands of patients. For samples of this magnitude a reasonable minimum subscale partition size might be hundreds of patients. For even larger training samples, it might be thousands of patients. These considerations will be revisited in section 5.

When training samples are sufficiently large, an additional subscale and corresponding training subsample added to account for missing observations may be further subdivided to improve accuracy. Such partitioning into sub-subscales and corresponding sub-subsamples is generally performed by means of a routinely recorded patient attribute or index, other than the stratifying attribute or index, that also appears to exert a large impact on the focal state or event. If the attribute or index with the greatest impact is used for stratification, the attribute or index with the second-greatest impact on the focal state or event might be used to make further subdivisions. Appendix A illustrates the subdivision procedure. Missing observations on mitotic rate are partitioned according to tumor thickness, improving, thereby, the accuracy of predicting disease-specific death within five years of melanoma diagnosis.

Constructing UIRI values for Cox regression is somewhat more complicated. The proportional hazards model underlying Cox regression defines proper spacing in terms of relative risks (hazard ratios). Thus, UIRI values must be assigned to partitioned subscales in such a way as to capture these ratios.

Defining zero-one dummy variables in the following manner and using them as independent variables in a Cox regression analysis will accomplish the desired result.

1. Count the number, N, of raw measurement scale partitions (subscales) produced in section 2.6. The count includes an extra partition for missing observations if any exist. N is always at least 2. [Clarifying comment: higher-valued partitions are assumed in this discussion to indicate higher levels of risk relative to experiencing the focal event.]

2. In the absence of missing observations, define a zero-one dummy variable for each of the N - 1 scale partitions, excluding the lowest-valued partition.

3. Each of the N - 1 partition-related dummy variables assigns a value of 1 to a patient in the total training sample if that patient's raw factor value falls in the associated partition (factor subscale). Otherwise, the partition-related dummy variable assigns a value of 0 to that patient.

4. By this procedure, all patients in the subsample associated with the lowest-valued partition will be assigned 0 values on all N - 1 dummy variables. All other patients will be assigned a value of 1 on exactly one of the N - 1 dummy variables and a value of 0 on all other dummy variables.

5. If an extra scale partition has been defined for missing observations, define a zero-one dummy variable for each of the N - 1 nonmissing scale partitions, including the lowest-valued partition.

6. Each of the N - 1 partition-related dummy variables assigns a value of 1 to a patient in the total training sample if that patient's raw factor value falls in the associated partition (factor subscale). Otherwise, the partition-related dummy variable assigns a value of 0 to that patient (including to a patient with a missing observation).

7. By this procedure, all patients in the subsample with a missing observation on the prognostic factor being considered will be assigned 0 values on all N - 1 dummy variables. All other patients will be assigned a value of 1 on exactly one of the N - 1 dummy variables and a value of 0 on all other dummy variables.

8. Whichever procedure is followed, dummy variables identify to which of the N scale partitions each patient in the total training sample belongs relative to the prognostic factor currently being considered.

9. Perform a Cox regression analysis. Use elapsed time until occurrence of the focal event (e.g., disease-specific death) as the dependent variable. Use the N - 1 zero-one dummy variables as independent variables. For illustrative purposes, assume an increasing risk factor.

10. Inspect the printed table of Cox regression results—one row for each of the N - 1 dummy variables. Identify the column of estimated relative risks (hazard ratios) in the printed table indicating increasing risk.

11. If there are no missing observations, assign (by convention) a relative risk of 1.0 to the lowest-valued partition (subscale) for which no dummy variable was defined. Then, assign an impact-reflecting index (UIRI) value to each of the N partitions (subscales) as the natural logarithm of its relative risk. This assigns a UIRI value of 0.0 (by convention) to the lowest-valued partition. Successively higher-valued partitions will be assigned successively higher-valued UIRI numbers.

12. If an extra scale partition has been defined for missing observations,

assign (by convention) a relative risk of 1.0 to the
missing-observation partition (subscale) for which no dummy variable
was defined. Identify the smallest relative risk. Then, rescale all
relative risks by dividing each by the smallest. Finally, assign a UIRI
value to each of the N partitions (subscales) as the natural logarithm
of its rescaled relative risk. Once again, this procedure will assign
(by convention) a UIRI value of 0.0 to the lowest-valued partition and
successively higher-valued UIRI numbers to higher-valued partitions.

Thus, in the case of Cox regression, UIRI values are calculated as the natural
logarithms of the relative risks (hazard ratios) associated with the N
partitions (subscales) of any given prognostic factor.

The interested reader is referred to appendix A for an annotated illustration
of the procedures and calculations outlined in sections 2.6 and 2.7.
Disease-specific death is selected as the focal event. The raw measurement
scale of mitotic rate as a prognostic factor is partitioned. UIRI values are
then produced for our sample of 1,222 melanoma patients—first for logistic
regression (five-year disease-specific death), and then for Cox regression
(elapsed time from initial diagnosis until disease-specific death). Individual
patient predictions are produced by both analyses and compared. Prognostic
accuracy is also assessed and compared.

2.8 Weighting Impact-Reflecting Index (UIRI) Values across Prognostic Factors

Applying the admissibility requirements outlined in section 2.5 and executing
the procedures outlined in sections 2.6 and 2.7 (illustrated in appendix A)
serve to preprocess all raw data. When stratified by risk group, as outlined in
section 2.4, these preprocessing steps are repeated for each risk group
separately. The result is as many tables of UIRI numbers as there are separate
risk groups.

Each table contains as many impact-reflecting indexes as there are prognostic
factors specifically admissible for the corresponding risk group. Each table
may be regarded as containing prognostic factor data for a separate training
sample. Separate analytical results can subsequently be merged, as will be
described in section 2.9.

After preprocessing, each UIRI value in each table purports to reflect both the
direction and the magnitude of the impact of its associated prognostic factor
on the focal event. Direction and magnitude of impact are encapsulated in the
numeric index values. Because there are no missing observations in any table,
each patient possesses a UIRI value on each admissible prognostic factor.

Raw prognostic data may be collected on many different scales. These raw
measurement scales may be highly disparate. Conveniently, however,
preprocessing guarantees that all numeric UIRI values in each table are
normalized. By construction, they are all on the same numeric scale. For this
reason, the relative prognostic potency of separate factors can be assessed by
estimating additive weights from their UIRI values.

Attempting to compare, strictly visually, odds ratios in logistic regression
and hazard ratios in Cox regression without prior PCM conversion to UIRIs is
quite challenging. The underlying factor scales can be confusingly disparate.

Additive factor weights may be calculated for logistic regression as follows.

1. Begin with a table of preprocessed UIRI values for some training sample of patients prepared to predict a dichotomous focal event.
2. Suppose that the table contains M rows, one for each patient in the sample, and N columns, one to hold UIRI numbers for each admissible prognostic factor.
3. There are no missing observations, so the table contains the product of M times N UIRI numbers.
4. The task is to identify a set of N nonnegative proportional weights adding to 1.0 that reflect the relative predictive potency of the N admissible prognostic factors. Once identified, the N weights can be used to construct a weighted average impact-reflecting index.
5. If all N factors were equally potent, then each weight would be 1/N, and their weighted average would be identical to their simple, unweighted average. However, if they differ in relative potency, they should receive different weights, and their weighted average would, typically, differ from their unweighted average.
6. Disease-specific death within five years of initial diagnosis has been chosen as the focal event in our patient-centered analysis. Therefore, weights should be selected to render the weighted average of the N component individual prediction probabilities (embodied, respectively, in the N impact-reflecting indexes) as close as possible to each patient's actual zero-one five-year disease-specific death outcome.
7. Minimizing the sum of the squared deviations is a convenient way to accomplish this.
8. A quadratic minimization problem based on nonnegative weights and a single linear constraint (the weights must add exactly to 1.0) has just been defined.
9. The Kuhn-Tucker conditions provide a necessary and sufficient mathematical solution to such a problem. From these, a workable solution procedure has been devised and reduced to computer code.
10. Applying this procedure to our sample of 1,222 melanoma patients resulted in the table of prognostic factor weights presented in appendix C. Applying the same procedure to our sample of 1,225 breast cancer patients resulted in the table of prognostic factor weights presented in appendix E.

Please note that the weights we have just calculated via least-squares are strictly for descriptive purposes. We have not suddenly abandoned the maximum likelihood estimation criterion underlying both logistic and Cox regression in favor of a sum-of-squared-deviations minimizing criterion. Logistic and Cox regression are still the preferred analytical procedures. Their output is still used to assess the accuracy of all individual patient predictions. For many people, however, these least-squares weights are simply easier to comprehend, intuitively, and to interpret than the corresponding coefficients generated by regression analysis. The weights should be viewed as nothing more than a descriptive adjunct to standard logistic and Cox regression output—a more understandable way to convey the concept of relative predictive potency.

2.9 Merging Separate Risk Groups and Incorporating Nontraditional Factors

As outlined in section 2.4, patients in both our melanoma and our breast cancer training samples were stratified by risk group prior to preprocessing their raw prognostic factor data. Completely separate analyses were then performed on the separate risk groups (training subsamples). These produced separate prognostic algorithms for each risk group in both cancers.

Merging separate risk group results means defining a composite, conditional, prognostic algorithm, which can be accomplished through the following steps.

1. The risk group membership of a targeted individual patient is first determined.
2. An appropriate prognostic algorithm is then selected for that patient from a fixed set of preconstructed algorithms—one for each predefined risk group.
3. In this manner, the concept of being similar to a targeted patient is operationally defined as belonging to that same patient's predefined risk group.
4. Preconstructing prognostic algorithms requires quite large collections of patient records. Updating and maintaining such records over time requires a currently nonexistent, ongoing infrastructure.
5. We believe that the practical value of our patient-centered methodology would be substantially enhanced by the existence of just such an ongoing infrastructure. These ideas will be revisited in section 5.

A traditional prognostic analysis was initially performed using the base case prognostic factors. Section 2.3 outlined six traditional (currently routinely recorded) prognostic factors for melanoma. Five of these were applicable, as well, to breast cancer and were used as its factor-centered base case.

The patient-centered procedural modifications incorporated in PCM served to improve the accuracy of individually tailored patient predictions in both base case analyses, when compared to traditional, nonmodified, factor-centered prognostic procedures. This will be shown in detail in section 3 for our 1,222 melanoma patients. It will be shown in detail in section 4 for our 1,225 breast cancer patients.

The news gets better. Since accuracy improvements were obtained compared to both factor-centered base case analyses, the same patient-centered modifications were applied to the analysis of nontraditional prognostic factors. Results were combined to produce composite prognostic algorithms reflecting the joint impact of both types of factors. Sections 3 and 4 will show how the addition of nontraditional prognostic factors to the base case improves still further the accuracy of individual patient predictions in both melanoma and breast cancer.

Assessing the efficacy of the patient-centered methodology constitutes our final task. It is accomplished by applying the individually tailored measures of prognostic accuracy introduced in section 2.2 to predictions made by the most comprehensive composite algorithm.

A simplified illustration of the assessment procedure is presented in appendix A. Each tailored measure is first applied to predictions based on a single prognostic factor (mitotic rate within a primary melanoma tumor). A computerized algorithm to generate the appropriate UIRI index for mitotic rate is executed. This is the Scale Partitioning and Spacing Algorithm (SPSA).

A more complete assessment is presented for melanoma patients in section 3 and appendixes B and C. A more complete assessment is presented for breast cancer patients in section 4 and appendixes D and E.

2.10 Statistical Consequences of an Altered Focus and Novel Success Measures

Section 1.3 set forth the altered focus of PCM compared to traditional, factor-centered methodology. The ultimate goal of PCM is to draw separately tailored conclusions about individual patients relative to a focal end point. Assessing the predictive potency of various prognostic factors in stratified patient populations regularly occurs along the way. However, such activities are penultimate. They are undertaken to facilitate PCM's ultimate objective.

This changes the fundamental nature of the questions we ask, the hypotheses we formulate and test, and the way we measure success. Such changes are immediate consequences of PCM's altered focus.

Toward this end, a number of procedural modifications to traditional analyses have already been outlined. Section 2.2 also suggested four substitute measures of predictive success. All four relate to the accuracy of individually tailored probabilistic predictions. Can PCM improve prognostic accuracy? That is the overarching question. The relevant hypotheses to formulate and test concern whether or not and the extent to which PCM is successful in making accuracy improvements compared to alternative methodologies.

Several statistical and presentational conventions will be followed throughout the remainder of this book. These conventions and the reasons for adopting them are explained below.

1. The principal measure of predictive accuracy will be AUC. This is the Area Under the Curve of a Receiver-Operating-Characteristic (ROC) analysis.

   AUC is a widely understood concept in medical research. Dr. Ware identified it as the usual measure of performance of a prognostic test. When two or more alternative methodologies generate probabilistic predictions of some focal event, a separate AUC will be estimated from the set of individually tailored probabilities produced by each methodology. These AUC values will be treated as descriptive statistics and compared accordingly.

   AUC values range from 0.0 to 1.0. Higher AUC values generally indicate more accurate predictions. An AUC of 0.0 designates no predictive accuracy, while an AUC of 1.0 designates maximum achievable accuracy.

   AUC values may also be augmented by the maximum number or percentage of correct predictions, as defined in section 2.2.

2. Whether or not one methodology produces more accurate predictions than another will be tested, statistically, by matched-sample comparisons. Each sample will contain the set of individually tailored probabilistic predictions assigned by a particular methodology to each patient in a training sample.

   Matching occurs patient-by-patient. Alternative methodologies assign separate focal event probabilities to each patient.

   When two methodologies are being compared, a matched-pairs statistical test (e.g., a matched-pairs T test; a Wilcoxon matched-pairs, signed-ranks test; or a binomial sign test) will be employed. When more than two are being compared, a statistical test involving matched n-tuples will be employed [e.g., a two-way analysis of variance (randomized block design) or a Friedman two-way analysis of variance by ranks].

In all such statistical tests, the uniform null hypothesis will be that no difference in predictive accuracy exists between or among alternative methodologies.

Formal hypothesis tests will generally be nondirectional (i.e., two-tail tests). It is the existence versus nonexistence of any systematic difference in accuracy that is being tested.

3. The direction and magnitude of differences in predictive accuracy will be measured by the absolute value of probabilistic prediction errors. A prediction error is the difference between whatever probability some methodology assigns to a patient that the focal event will occur and its 0/1 actual occurrence, where zero signifies nonoccurrence and one signifies occurrence. The more accurate methodology is then the one that generates systematically smaller absolute-error differences.

Using probabilistic errors to quantify predictive accuracy can introduce outliers (i.e., extreme values) into the analysis. When a patient actually experiences a rare focal event, the difference between that patient's (typically close to zero) assigned probability and the 1.0 signifying actual occurrence can be much larger than the error differences assigned to the many other patients who do not experience it. Outliers can also arise, although in the reverse manner, with very frequently occurring focal events.

The incidence of outliers complicates the determination of systematically smaller or larger error differences, when means are calculated and compared. It can also undermine the presumption of normally distributed test statistics underlying many parametric procedures (e.g., the analysis of variance and T tests).

Via the magic of the Central Limit Theorem, the problem of outliers is reduced as sample sizes increase. It will sometimes be necessary, however, to assess the direction and magnitude of differences in predictive accuracy by comparing samples of small to intermediate size.

The Wilcoxon matched-pairs, signed-ranks test is less sensitive to outliers than the parametric matched-pairs T test. It is based on mean differences in the ranks of matched-pair differences rather than on mean differences between each pair of probabilities, which might include outliers. So also, and for the same reason is the Friedman two-way analysis of variance by ranks less sensitive than the parametric analysis of variance (randomized block design). The binomial sign test is not at all sensitive to outliers when performing a matched-pairs comparison.

Both the Wilcoxon test and the Friedman test have very high relative efficiency (in the neighborhood of 95 percent) in their ability to reject the null hypothesis. Hence, very little needs to be sacrificed to protect effectively against troublesome outliers.

These nonparametric tests will be regularly performed throughout the book. Occasionally, their slightly more powerful equivalent parametric tests will also be performed and reported—especially when sample sizes are quite adequate.

4. That the binomial sign test is insensitive to outliers suggests a uniform way to calibrate both the direction and the magnitude of predictive accuracy when comparing different methodologies.

   Relative predictive accuracy can be encapsulated in an index of error reduction. The index is designed to resemble an ordinary correlation coefficient. It is the signed proportion of net error reductions in any set of matched-pair comparisons, calculated as follows.

   a. First, select one of two methodologies as more likely to make accurate predictions (e.g., by comparing estimated AUC values).
   b. Then, count the number of matched pairs wherein the selected methodology generates the smaller absolute probabilistic prediction error. These are labeled error reductions.
   c. Subtract from this the number of matched pairs wherein the selected methodology generates the larger absolute error. These are labeled error increases.
   d. Ignore matched pairs with equal absolute errors.
   e. Finally, divide the difference between these two counts by their sum (i.e., the number of matched pairs containing nonidentical absolute errors).

   The index ranges in value from −1.0, when all comparisons produce (unanticipated) error increases, to +1.0, when all comparisons produce (anticipated) error reductions. As with a correlation coefficient, it has a value of 0.0 when the number of error reductions is exactly offset by an equal number of error increases.

5. The index of error reduction can be calculated for any set of matched prediction errors. Its sign and magnitude indicate which of any two methodologies generates the more accurate probabilistic predictions.

   Since it is normalized to fall between −1.0 and +1.0, the relative predictive accuracy of several different methodologies may be determined at a glance. Alternative methodologies may then be ordered according to their relative predictive accuracy.

6. The distribution of the Wilcoxon test statistic rapidly approaches normality as the number of nontied matched-pair comparisons increases. Whenever the count exceeds twenty-five, this approximation becomes quite satisfactory. Hence, an equivalent standardized Z statistic will generally be computed and referred to the unit normal distribution for statistical significance testing. The Z statistic is the Wilcoxon test statistic divided by its standard deviation. Only for small counts (twenty-five or fewer nontied matched pairs) will an exact probability be computed for Wilcoxon p values.

7. PCM has been specifically designed to anticipate large amounts of missing patient data. No patient record is required to possess complete data on all prognostic factors. The SPSA algorithm assigns particular numeric values to every missing observation. This can introduce a substantial number of tied observation values into the data being analyzed, which, in turn, can also skew or otherwise undermine the presumption of normally distributed test statistics.

   The Wilcoxon and binomial sign tests eliminate within-pair tied observations. The Kruskal-Wallis test, the Mann-Whitney test, and both the Spearman and Kendall rank correlation tests contain explicit procedures that correct for tied observations. Their parametric

equivalents lack such procedures and, typically, assume normal
distributions.

These considerations constitute a second reason to systematically
substitute nonparametric for parametric statistical tests in assessing
PCM.

8. The design of PCM renders it especially vulnerable to overfitting a
prognostic algorithm to training data. The same devices that PCM
employs to improve predictive accuracy can also produce this unwanted
side effect. The nature and seriousness of overfitting will be
discussed in some detail in section 5.

Unless otherwise indicated, all applications of the SPSA algorithm will
be executed with a minimum scale partition size of twenty-five patient
observations. This will provide some protection against excessive
overfitting. Larger minimum scale partition sizes afford greater
protection and will occasionally be adopted.

3.0 APPLYING PCM TO 1,222 MELANOMA PATIENTS

As stated in section 2.1, disease-specific death within five years following initial diagnosis has been chosen as the focal event to be predicted, probabilistically, by our proposed patient-centered methodology.

A sample of 1,222 patients diagnosed with cutaneous melanoma between July 1971 and November 2006 by the University of California at San Francisco (UCSF) was collected and analyzed to illustrate PCM. These patients were followed up until October 2010. Median and mean follow-up periods were 7.44 and 7.93 years, respectively. Selected attributes of this melanoma training sample are presented in appendix B.

AJCC stage at diagnosis was determined for most (83.4 percent) of the 1,222 patients. Tumor thickness and AJCC T stage (T1, T2, T3, or T4) were determined for the remainder (16.6 percent).

All 1,222 patients either died of metastatic melanoma within five years of diagnosis or survived for more than five years. The following table shows that 281 of the 1,222 (23.0 percent) suffered disease-specific death within five years, while the other 941 patients (77.0 percent) did not.

VALUE OF DEFINING EXPRESSION	VALUE OF ATTRIBUTE DSS5YR		
	DSS>5YRS	MM DEATH=<5YRS	TOTAL
MELANOMA DEATH=<5 YRS.	0	281	281
MELANOMA DEATH>5 YRS.	128	0	128
NO MELANOMA DEATH, F/U>5 YRS.	813	0	813
TOTAL	941	281	1222

Notes: MM DEATH means death due to metastatic melanoma. F/U means follow-up period in years. DSS means disease-specific survival.

Accuracy in predicting an individual patient's disease-specific death within five years following initial diagnosis is improved by:

1. first stratifying patients according to their risk of experiencing the focal event, as indicated by their AJCC stage at time of diagnosis;
2. then executing the SPSA algorithm—separately within each risk subgroup—to transform each traditional (i.e., routinely recorded) base case prognostic factor into a corresponding UIRI;
3. then adding nontraditional prognostic factors—transformed to corresponding UIRIs by the same SPSA algorithm applied, separately, to each risk subgroup;
4. then performing a separate logistic regression analysis within each risk subgroup, using transformed UIRI indexes as inputs (independent variables); and
5. merging the results obtained from each risk subgroup's logistic regression analysis into a composite, individual prediction algorithm.

It will be instructive to see how successive steps in this sequence provide incremental improvements in accuracy.

3.1 Stratifying Patients into Low-Risk, Medium-Risk, and High-Risk Subgroups

The first task was to stratify the 1,222 patients into appropriate subgroups.

Among the widely understood and routinely recorded traditional prognostic factors in melanoma, AJCC stage and tumor thickness are generally regarded as the best single predictors of MM death. We verified this for our 1,222-patient training sample by selecting the subset of 849 patients with no missing observations on any candidate factors and by then:

1. executing a dummy-variable logistic regression analysis, using the AJCC staging categories (i.e., 1a, 1b, 2a, etc.) as independent variables;
2. assigning estimated five-year MM death probabilities to each staging category according to the calculations outlined in section 2.2; and
3. applying SPSA to the other six traditional factors identified by the AJCC, with a uniformly specified minimum partition size of 150 patients to guarantee highly stable five-year MM death probability estimates.

The probabilities estimated for each AJCC stage at diagnosis and the resulting six UIRIs were then used as seven independent variables in a multivariate logistic regression analysis.

AJCC stage, tumor thickness, and mitotic rate were the only three statistically significant prognostic factors in the multivariate analysis. AJCC stage at diagnosis was the most significant of the three, with an associated two-tail p value less than 0.00005. Mitotic rate was almost as significant. Tumor thickness was much less significant (two-tail p value between 0.01 and 0.02).

Recalling Dr. Ware's admonition that statistical significance alone does not guarantee accurate predictions at the individual patient level, we compared the absolute-value probabilistic prediction errors for these three factors. Both a randomized blocks two-way analysis of variance and its corresponding nonparametric Friedman test were performed to ascertain their relative predictive accuracies.

The Friedman test was performed to confirm that the results of the corresponding parametric two-way analysis of variance were not compromised by outliers, by the presence of numerous tied prediction error differences, or by any other serious distributional anomalies in the data.

An edited computer printout of both test results is shown in the immediately following paragraphs. Separate rankings of the three absolute-value prediction errors were made for each of the 849 patients in the Friedman test, where lower ranks signify smaller absolute-value prediction errors.

There are 849 matched 3-tuples possessing completely defined data. This is sufficient both for a randomized blocks two-way analysis of variance and for its corresponding nonparametric equivalent Friedman two-way analysis of variance by ranks.

A randomized blocks two-way analysis of variance (ANOVA) has been performed.

The mean value of AJCC STAGE error in each matched 3-tuple is .2888.
The mean value of TUMOR THICKNESS error in each matched 3-tuple is .3119.
The mean value of MITOTIC RATE error in each matched 3-tuple is .3151.

The 849 matched 3-tuples display an *EXTREMELY SIGNIFICANT DEPARTURE* from what would be expected under the nondirectional randomized blocks two-way analysis of variance if the sample of 849 AJCC STAGE error values, the sample of 849 TUMOR THICKNESS error values, and the sample of 849 MITOTIC RATE error values had all been drawn from the same normally distributed population, or if they had been drawn, respectively, from 3 identical, normally distributed populations.

Analysis of variance significance test result: p value is 0.0000.

A Friedman two-way analysis of variance by ranks has been performed.

The average rank of AJCC STAGE error in each matched 3-tuple is 1.8198.
The average rank of TUMOR THICKNESS error in each matched 3-tuple is 2.0318.
The average rank of MITOTIC RATE error in each matched 3-tuple is 2.1484.

The 849 matched 3-tuples display an *EXTREMELY SIGNIFICANT DEPARTURE* from what would be expected under the nondirectional Friedman analysis if the sample of 849 AJCC STAGE error ranks, the sample of 849 TUMOR THICKNESS error ranks, and the sample of 849 MITOTIC RATE error ranks had all been drawn from the same population, or if they had been drawn, respectively, from 3 identically distributed populations of absolute error rank numbers.

Friedman significance test result: p value is 0.0000.

Note the dramatic difference between the relative (multivariate) statistical significance of the three prognostic factors and their relative (univariate) predictive accuracy. Dr. Ware's admonition appears to be quite well-founded.

A matched-pairs T test and its corresponding nonparametric Wilcoxon matched-pairs, signed-ranks test and its corresponding binomial sign test were also performed on the matched (by patient) differences in absolute probabilistic prediction errors. Absolute errors were generated both for AJCC stage and for tumor thickness. These tests resulted in a T value of 4.30, significant at a two-tail p value less than 0.00005; a corresponding Wilcoxon difference, significant at a two-tail p value less than 0.00005; and a corresponding binomial sign difference, significant at a two-tail p value of 0.0005. An index of error reduction = 0.1213 and all three statistical tests confirmed AJCC stage at diagnosis as the most accurate single predictor.

The nonparametric Wilcoxon and sign test results once again indicated that the results of the matched-pairs T test were not compromised by the presence of outliers, tied prediction error differences, or any other serious distributional anomalies in the data—at least not in this large a sample.

Consequently, the PCM criteria suggested stratifying our 1,222 patients into risk subgroups based on their initial AJCC stage. When complete AJCC stage is indeterminate, patients can then be stratified according to their T stage.

The dummy-variable logistic regression analysis (see section 3.2 for details) exposed two risk inversions in the staging categories among these 849 patients.

1. The forty-five stage 3a patients experienced a 22.22 percent incidence of MM death within five years, while the ninety-one stage 2b patients experienced a 24.18 percent incidence.
2. The fifty-eight stage 2c patients experienced a 37.93 percent incidence of MM death within five years, while the forty-five stage 3a patients experienced a 22.22 percent incidence, the 118 stage 3b patients experienced a 31.36 percent incidence, and the 128 stage 3c patients experienced a 56.25 percent incidence.

The first of these two inversions was statistically insignificant. The inversion between stage 2c and 3a incidences was somewhat significant [both T test and Mann-Whitney test (corrected for tied observations) one-tail p values were 0.04]. It suggested grouping together stage 2b and 3a patients and placing stage 2c patients into a higher risk subgroup than the other stage 2 patients.

Additional trial-and-error analyses led to the following stratification.

1. The low-risk subgroup consisted of 503 patients initially diagnosed with stage 1a (78) or 1b (322) melanoma, plus 103 T1 patients, collectively experiencing a 5.37 percent incidence of MM death within five years.
2. The medium-risk subgroup consisted of 423 patients initially diagnosed with stage 2a (105) or 2b (94) or 3a (51) or 3b (138) melanoma, plus two nodally involved T1 patients and thirty-three T2 patients, experiencing a 24.59 percent incidence of MM death within five years.
3. The high-risk subgroup consisted of 296 patients initially diagnosed with stage 2c (63) or 3c (161) or 4 (7) melanoma, plus twenty-eight T3 patients and thirty-seven T4 patients, experiencing a 50.68 percent incidence of MM death within five years.

Stratifying the total sample into these three risk subgroups served to maintain sufficient subgroup sizes to support stable statistical estimates, while producing an incidence rank order consistent both with the incidences of MM death within five years of diagnosis within our training sample and with the five-year DSS survival rates by initial stage reported in 2001 by the AJCC on a sample of more than ten thousand worldwide melanoma patients.

The dramatic between-subgroup differences in the incidence of death due to metastatic melanoma were highly significant when assessed by a Kruskal-Wallis test corrected for tied observations (two-tail p value < 0.00005), as were the differences in DSS survival rates when assessed by Kaplan-Meier analysis (Log-rank test two-tail p value < 0.0001, Figure 1).

3.2   Analysis of Traditional Prognostic Factors without Missing Observations

Now let us adopt as a factor-centered base case the six AJCC routinely recorded prognostic factors, exactly as defined by the AJCC for 2010 and beyond. All six factors and initial AJCC stage at diagnosis were defined for 849 of the 1,222 melanoma patients. In a typical factor-centered approach, patients with any missing observations are deleted from the analysis, and those with complete data are not stratified according to their risk of experiencing the focal event. The results of a standard, factor-centered logistic regression on these six prognostic factors with no missing observations are shown directly below.

RESULTS OF LOGISTIC REGRESSION ANALYSIS (LINEAR MODEL)

The dependent variable is a binary-coded numeric variable whose values are either 0 or 1. It is embodied in the first expression (parameter) of the LOGREG command, which is just the attribute DSSDUMMY.

The independent variable AJCCAGE is just the attribute AJCCAGE.
The independent variable AJCCSEX is just the attribute AJCCSEX.
The independent variable AJCCSITE is just the attribute AJCCSITE.
The independent variable AJCCTHIC is just the attribute AJCCTHIC.
The independent variable AJCCMITR is just the attribute AJCCMITR.
The independent variable AJCCULC is just the attribute AJCCULC.

Figure 1

Kaplan-Meier Survival Analysis

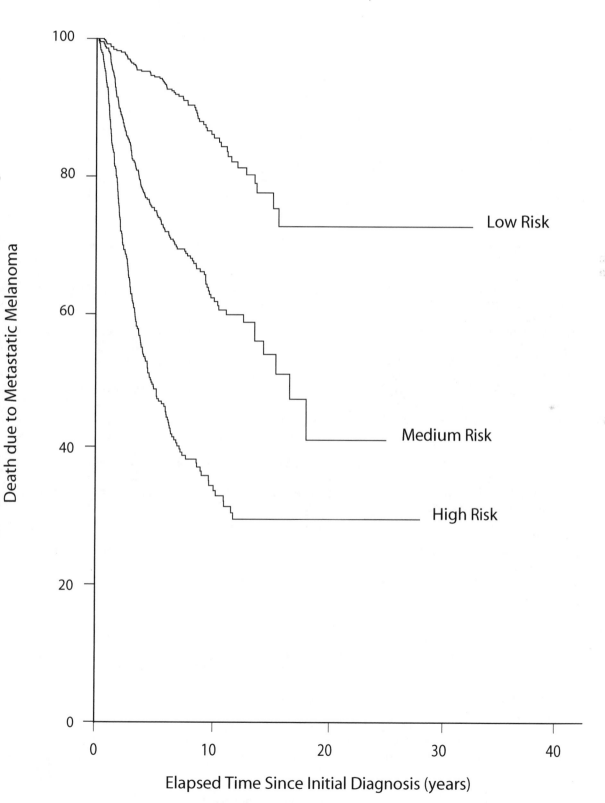

Likelihood ratio chi-square statistic: 132.946, two-tail p value: .0000 (based on 6 degrees of freedom and 849 complete observations).

INDEPENDENT VARIABLE	REGRESSION COEFFICIENT	STANDARD DEVIATION	CHI-SQUARE (DF = 1)	2-TAIL P VALUE	ODDS RATIO MULTIPLIER
intercept	-3.9654	.6057	42.8533	.0000	.0190
AJCCAGE	-.0094	.0569	.0272	.8689	.9907
AJCCSEX	.2681	.1952	1.8872	.1695	1.3075
AJCCSITE	.2624	.1944	1.8213	.1772	1.3000
AJCCTHIC	.6865	.0973	49.8223	.0000	1.9867
AJCCMITR	.2651	.5522	.2305	.6312	1.3036
AJCCULC	.7833	.1869	17.5730	.0000	2.1887

GOODNESS OF STATISTICAL FIT OF LOGISTIC REGRESSION MODEL

Pearson chi-square fit statistic (based on 204 degrees of freedom): 210.068, p value: .3705.

Deviance chi-square fit statistic (based on 204 degrees of freedom): 196.937, p value: .6258.

[Technical note: One might wonder why mitotic rate (AJCCMITR) appears in the above table to be a statistically insignificant predictor of MM death when it was reported in section 3.1 as being so significant in the multivariate logistic regression analysis of the same 849 patients. The answer is twofold. First, AJCC stage is not one of the independent variables in this regression. It was the single most potent predictor in section 3.1. Second, all independent variables in this regression are the preprocessed transformations of raw data recommended by the AJCC for 2010 and beyond. All independent variables in the regression analysis reported in section 3.1 were transformed into UIRI values, preprocessed by SPSA. Not transforming mitotic rate into a UIRI via SPSA, but merely dichotomizing it into AJCCMITR, had a huge impact.]

The attribute definition that immediately follows this and all subsequent displays of logistic regression output implements the prognostic algorithm presented in section 2.2. Thus, CN5YRDPR implements the prognostic algorithm for the traditional factor-centered base case analysis.

DEFINE CN5YRDPR:
EXP(-3.9654-.0094*AJCCAGE+.2681*AJCCSEX+.2624*AJCCSITE+.6865*AJCCTHIC+
.2651*AJCCMITR+.7833*AJCCULC)/[1+
EXP(-3.9654-.0094*AJCCAGE+.2681*AJCCSEX+.2624*AJCCSITE+.6865*AJCCTHIC+
.2651*AJCCMITR+.7833*AJCCULC)] IF FIRSTAGE#UNDEFS

The CN5YRDPR attribute assigns an individual probability of experiencing death due to metastatic melanoma within five years of diagnosis to each of the 849 patients based on the above six AJCC traditional prognostic factors. These 849 individual probabilities were then subjected to a ROC/AUC analysis.

The area under the complete ROC curve was estimated to be 0.7593.

The next analysis we shall refer to as the practice-centered base case. So labeling it recognizes that many practicing physicians consider initial AJCC stage as the generally accepted basis for making individual patient prognoses.

Since AJCC stage is a classification index, the practice-centered base case analysis was a logistic regression based on dummy variables. As usual, the dependent variable was MM death within five years of diagnosis. The independent variables were zero-one dummy variables identifying, respectively, in which stage each patient was initially diagnosed. By transforming the output into probabilities, an individually tailored probabilistic prediction was made for each patient. Predictions were based on initial AJCC stage alone. There were no missing observations included in this practice-centered base case analysis. The mechanics of dummy-variable logistic regression analysis, in combination with the prognostic algorithm, produced a pleasantly familiar result. The probability of MM death within five years assigned to each of the 849 patients was its incidence among all patients classified in that patient's same initial AJCC stage. It is common practice to use incidence by stage as a patient prediction when nothing else is available to make an individualized prognosis.

RESULTS OF LOGISTIC REGRESSION ANALYSIS (LINEAR MODEL)

The dependent variable is a binary-coded numeric variable whose values are either 0 or 1. It is embodied in the first expression (parameter) of the LOGREG command, which is just the attribute DSSDUMMY.

The independent variable EXPRESSION2 is 1 IF FIRSTAGE="1b" ELSE 0.
The independent variable EXPRESSION3 is 1 IF FIRSTAGE="2a" ELSE 0.
The independent variable EXPRESSION4 is 1 IF FIRSTAGE="2b" ELSE 0.
The independent variable EXPRESSION5 is 1 IF FIRSTAGE="2c" ELSE 0.
The independent variable EXPRESSION6 is 1 IF FIRSTAGE="3a" ELSE 0.
The independent variable EXPRESSION7 is 1 IF FIRSTAGE="3b" ELSE 0.
The independent variable EXPRESSION8 is 1 IF FIRSTAGE="3c" ELSE 0.

Likelihood ratio chi-square statistic: 156.333, two-tail p value: .0000 (based on 7 degrees of freedom and 843 complete observations).

INDEPENDENT VARIABLE	REGRESSION COEFFICIENT	STANDARD DEVIATION	CHI-SQUARE (DF = 1)	2-TAIL P VALUE	ODDS RATIO MULTIPLIER
intercept	−3.7842	1.0113	14.0019	.0002	.0227
EXPRESSION2	.9139	1.0480	.7605	.3832	2.4939
EXPRESSION3	2.1623	1.0477	4.2600	.0390	8.6914
EXPRESSION4	2.6411	1.0405	6.4429	.0111	14.0290
EXPRESSION5	3.2917	1.0469	9.8867	.0017	26.8889
EXPRESSION6	2.5314	1.0730	5.5660	.0183	12.5714
EXPRESSION7	3.0007	1.0306	8.4775	.0036	20.0988
EXPRESSION8	4.0355	1.0269	15.4440	.0001	56.5714

[Technical note: Seven zero-one dummy variables served as the independent variables. Patients diagnosed in stage 1a were assigned zero values on all seven dummy variables. Also, all six of the 849 patients initially diagnosed in stage 4 died within five years of metastatic melanoma. They were not included in this practice-centered base case logistic regression analysis.]

```
DEFINE CF5YRDPR:
EXP(-3.7842)/[1+EXP(-3.7842)] IF FIRSTAGE="1a" ELSE
EXP(-3.7842+.9139)/[1+EXP(-3.7842+.9139)] IF FIRSTAGE="1b" ELSE
EXP(-3.7842+2.1623)/[1+EXP(-3.7842+2.1623)] IF FIRSTAGE="2a" ELSE
EXP(-3.7842+2.6411)/[1+EXP(-3.7842+2.6411)] IF FIRSTAGE="2b" ELSE
EXP(-3.7842+3.2917)/[1+EXP(-3.7842+3.2917)] IF FIRSTAGE="2c" ELSE
EXP(-3.7842+2.5314)/[1+EXP(-3.7842+2.5314)] IF FIRSTAGE="3a" ELSE
EXP(-3.7842+3.0007)/[1+EXP(-3.7842+3.0007)] IF FIRSTAGE="3b" ELSE
EXP(-3.7842+4.0355)/[1+EXP(-3.7842+4.0355)] IF FIRSTAGE="3c" ELSE
1.0000 IF FIRSTAGE="4"
```

The CF5YRDPR attribute assigns an individual probability of experiencing death due to metastatic melanoma within five years of diagnosis to each of the 849 patients based solely on AJCC stage at diagnosis as a classificatory (dummy-variable) input to logistic regression. These 849 individual probabilities were then subjected to a ROC/AUC analysis.

The area under the complete ROC curve was estimated to be 0.7831.

Substituting the initial AJCC staging classification for the AJCC six traditional factors increased the AUC by 0.0238, from 0.7593 to 0.7831. It also produced an index of error reduction = 0.3310 compared to the factor-centered base case analysis. A Wilcoxon matched-pairs, signed-ranks test was performed on the 849 matched pairs of probabilistic prediction errors, resulting in a normalized Z statistic = 5.82, with a two-tail p value < 0.00005.

Each prognostic factor's optimal scale partitioning and numeric rescaling is embodied in its univariate impact-reflecting index (UIRI) produced by the Scale Partitioning and Spacing Algorithm (SPSA). The six UIRI indexes were substituted for their corresponding six AJCC traditional prognostic factors, and the following logistic regression analysis was performed.

RESULTS OF LOGISTIC REGRESSION ANALYSIS (LINEAR MODEL)

The dependent variable is a binary-coded numeric variable whose values are either 0 or 1. It is embodied in the first expression (parameter) of the LOGREG command, which is just the attribute DSSDUMMY.

The independent variable AGECUIRI is just the attribute AGECUIRI.
The independent variable SEXCUIRI is just the attribute SEXCUIRI.
The independent variable SITCUIRI is just the attribute SITCUIRI.
The independent variable THKCUIRI is just the attribute THKCUIRI.
The independent variable MITCUIRI is just the attribute MITCUIRI.
The independent variable ULCCUIRI is just the attribute ULCCUIRI.

Likelihood ratio chi-square statistic: 170.869, two-tail p value: .0000 (based on 6 degrees of freedom and 849 complete observations).

INDEPENDENT VARIABLE	REGRESSION COEFFICIENT	STANDARD DEVIATION	CHI-SQUARE (DF = 1)	2-TAIL P VALUE	ODDS RATIO MULTIPLIER
intercept	-6.5486	1.2586	27.0726	.0000	.0014
AGECUIRI	1.9769	1.7836	1.2285	.2677	7.2206
SEXCUIRI	4.4218	2.7536	2.5787	.1083	83.2455
SITCUIRI	6.0971	4.7149	1.6723	.1960	444.5858
THKCUIRI	3.7130	.6973	28.3529	.0000	40.9767
MITCUIRI	3.3260	.6676	24.8215	.0000	27.8259
ULCCUIRI	1.8577	.7715	5.7982	.0160	6.4091

GOODNESS OF STATISTICAL FIT OF LOGISTIC REGRESSION MODEL

Pearson chi-square fit statistic (based on 531 degrees of freedom): 518.217, p value: .6478.

Deviance chi-square fit statistic (based on 531 degrees of freedom): 510.037, p value: .7371.

```
DEFINE CA5YRDPR:
EXP(-6.5486+1.9769*AGECUIRI+4.4218*SEXCUIRI+6.0971*SITCUIRI+3.7130*THKCUIRI+
3.3260*MITCUIRI+1.8577*ULCCUIRI)/[1+
EXP(-6.5486+1.9769*AGECUIRI+4.4218*SEXCUIRI+6.0971*SITCUIRI+3.7130*THKCUIRI+
3.3260*MITCUIRI+1.8577*ULCCUIRI)] IF FIRSTAGE#UNDEFS
```

The CA5YRDPR attribute assigns an individual probability of experiencing death
due to metastatic melanoma within five years of diagnosis to each of the 849
patients based on the above six AJCC traditional prognostic factors converted
by SPSA to corresponding UIRI values, but without any consideration of AJCC
stage at diagnosis. These 849 individual probabilities were then subjected to a
ROC/AUC analysis.

The area under the complete ROC curve was estimated to be 0.7914.

Converting the six AJCC traditional prognostic factors to corresponding UIRI
values produced predictive improvements with respect to both base case
analyses. The improvement in AUC compared to the factor-centered base case was
0.0321, from 0.7593 to 0.7914. Compared to the practice-centered base case the
improvement in AUC was 0.0083, from 0.7831 to 0.7914. A Wilcoxon test performed
on the 849 matched pairs of probabilistic prediction errors generated an index
of error reduction = 0.2909 compared to the factor-centered base case, which
was statistically significant (two-tail p value < 0.00005). Compared to the
practice-centered base case, the improved AUC proved to be statistically
insignificant. Substituting the UIRI values as independent variables also
produced a somewhat better statistical fit with the logistic regression model.
Producing a better statistical fit will turn out to be a consistent advantage
of using UIRI values in logistic regression.

The last analysis to be performed with no missing observations was designed to
assess the incremental improvement in predictive accuracy realizable from
stratifying patients into low-risk, medium-risk, and high-risk subgroups—
given that the six UIRI indexes had been substituted for their corresponding
six AJCC traditional prognostic factors as independent variable inputs to
logistic regression. Three separate logistic regressions were executed, one on
each risk subgroup. This required executing SPSA three times to produce a UIRI
value for each of the six AJCC traditional prognostic factors, separately, for
each risk subgroup. To distinguish among them, AGELUIRI designated the UIRI for
AGE in the low-risk subgroup, AGEMUIRI designated the UIRI for AGE in the
medium-risk subgroup, and AGEHUIRI designated the UIRI for AGE in the high-risk
subgroup. L, M, and H designators were also used to distinguish UIRI values
among subgroups for the other five AJCC traditional prognostic factors.

All three regression analyses generated highly significant likelihood ratio
chi-square statistics. The three separate regression outputs are not shown
below, but the expression used to merge the three sets of results into the
definition of the CS5YRDPR attribute is displayed.

```
DEFINE CS5YRDPR:
EXP(-7.5232+22.8493*AGELUIRI+11.2673*SEXLUIRI+25.6214*SITLUIRI+
9.7513*THKLUIRI+13.8800*MITLUIRI)/[1+
EXP(-7.5232+22.8493*AGELUIRI+11.2673*SEXLUIRI+25.6214*SITLUIRI+
9.7513*THKLUIRI+13.8800*MITLUIRI)] IF
AJCCAGE#UNDEFN AND AJCCSEX#UNDEFN AND AJCCSITE#UNDEFN AND
AJCCTHIC#UNDEFN AND AJCCMITR#UNDEFN AND AJCCULC#UNDEFN AND
FIRSTAGE#UNDEFS AND RISKLEVL=LOWRISK ELSE
EXP(-7.4608+4.3682*AGEMUIRI+6.4231*SEXMUIRI+5.2013*SITMUIRI+
3.8302*THKMUIRI+4.7507*MITMUIRI+.9016*ULCMUIRI)/[1+
EXP(-7.4608+4.3682*AGEMUIRI+6.4231*SEXMUIRI+5.2013*SITMUIRI+
```

```
3.8302*THKMUIRI+4.7507*MITMUIRI+.9016*ULCMUIRI)] IF
AJCCAGE#UNDEFN AND AJCCSEX#UNDEFN AND AJCCSITE#UNDEFN AND
AJCCTHIC#UNDEFN AND AJCCMITR#UNDEFN AND AJCCULC#UNDEFN AND
FIRSTAGE#UNDEFS AND RISKLEVL=MEDRISK ELSE
EXP(-4.5823+2.4538*SEXHUIRI+3.9919*SITHUIRI+.8139*THKHUIRI+
4.1429*MITHUIRI-2.4449*ULCHUIRI)/[1+
EXP(-4.5823+2.4538*SEXHUIRI+3.9919*SITHUIRI+.8139*THKHUIRI+
4.1429*MITHUIRI-2.4449*ULCHUIRI)] IF
AJCCAGE#UNDEFN AND AJCCSEX#UNDEFN AND AJCCSITE#UNDEFN AND
AJCCTHIC#UNDEFN AND AJCCMITR#UNDEFN AND AJCCULC#UNDEFN AND
FIRSTAGE#UNDEFS AND RISKLEVL=HIGHRISK
```

The CS5YRDPR attribute assigns an individual probability of experiencing death due to metastatic melanoma within five years of diagnosis to each of the 849 patients based on the above six AJCC traditional prognostic factors converted by SPSA to corresponding UIRI values—separately for each risk subgroup—but without using AJCC stage as an independent variable of logistic regression. These 849 individual probabilities were then subjected to a ROC/AUC analysis.

The area under the complete ROC curve was estimated to be 0.8220.

Stratifying patients into low-risk, medium-risk, and high-risk subgroups and converting traditional prognostic factors to corresponding UIRI values improved predictive accuracy relative to all three previous analyses. It increased the AUC by 0.0306, from 0.7914 to 0.8220, compared to simply converting traditional prognostic factors to corresponding UIRI values, which generated the most accurate of the three previous predictions. It also produced an index of error reduction = 0.2812 compared to the same simple conversions. A Wilcoxon test was performed on the 849 matched pairs of probabilistic prediction errors, showing a normalized Z statistic = 8.41, with a two-tail p value < 0.00005.

These results show that the combined impact of stratifying patients by risk subgroup and then substituting corresponding UIRI values for the six AJCC traditional prognostic factors (separately by risk subgroup) produced significantly more accurate individual probabilistic predictions (in terms of both AUC values and probabilistic prediction errors) than basing predictions solely on initial AJCC staging classification. Because none of the 849 melanoma patients possessed any missing observations, these results cannot be attributed in any way to the somewhat unusual manner in which SPSA handles missing data.

3.3   Analysis of Traditional Prognostic Factors with Missing Observations

Once again, we adopted as a traditional factor-centered base case the six AJCC routinely recorded prognostic factors, exactly as defined by the AJCC for 2010 and beyond. Excluding patient sex, the other five traditional AJCC factors contained missing observations for at least some of the 1,222 melanoma patients.

Patients were not stratified according to their risk of experiencing disease-specific death within five years for this revised factor-centered base case analysis. What was different here was that no patients with missing observations were excluded. Instead, they were treated in a commonly practiced factor-centered manner. Each missing observation was replaced by the mean of the nonmissing observations for that prognostic factor in the training sample.

The results of a standard logistic regression on these six prognostic factors, with missing observations replaced by mean values, are shown on the next page.

```
DEFINE AJCCAGEM: AJCCAGE IF AJCCAGE#UNDEFN ELSE MEAN(AJCCAGE)
DEFINE AJCCSITM: AJCCSITE IF AJCCSITE#UNDEFN ELSE MEAN(AJCCSITE)
DEFINE AJCCTHKM: AJCCTHIC IF AJCCTHIC#UNDEFN ELSE MEAN(AJCCTHIC)
DEFINE AJCCMITM: AJCCMITR IF AJCCMITR#UNDEFN ELSE MEAN(AJCCMITR)
DEFINE AJCCULCM: AJCCULC IF AJCCULC#UNDEFN ELSE MEAN(AJCCULC)
```

RESULTS OF LOGISTIC REGRESSION ANALYSIS (LINEAR MODEL)

The dependent variable is a binary-coded numeric variable whose values are
either 0 or 1. It is embodied in the first expression (parameter) of the LOGREG
command, which is just the attribute DSSDUMMY.

The independent variable AJCCAGEM is just the attribute AJCCAGEM.
The independent variable AJCCSEX is just the attribute AJCCSEX.
The independent variable AJCCSITM is just the attribute AJCCSITM.
The independent variable AJCCTHKM is just the attribute AJCCTHKM.
The independent variable AJCCMITM is just the attribute AJCCMITM.
The independent variable AJCCULCM is just the attribute AJCCULCM.

Likelihood ratio chi-square statistic: 193.665, two-tail p value: .0000 (based
on 6 degrees of freedom and 1222 complete observations).

INDEPENDENT VARIABLE	REGRESSION COEFFICIENT	STANDARD DEVIATION	CHI-SQUARE (DF = 1)	2-TAIL P VALUE	ODDS RATIO MULTIPLIER
intercept	-3.8897	.5167	56.6769	.0000	.0205
AJCCAGEM	.0140	.0473	.0878	.7669	1.0141
AJCCSEX	.2844	.1628	3.0489	.0808	1.3289
AJCCSITM	.1840	.1616	1.2965	.2549	1.2020
AJCCTHKM	.7126	.0744	91.6103	.0000	2.0392
AJCCMITM	.1785	.4822	.1370	.7112	1.1954
AJCCULCM	.6932	.1664	17.3562	.0000	2.0001

GOODNESS OF STATISTICAL FIT OF LOGISTIC REGRESSION MODEL

Pearson chi-square fit statistic (based on 388 degrees of freedom): 415.196,
p value: .1640.

Deviance chi-square fit statistic (based on 388 degrees of freedom): 405.037,
p value: .2654.

```
DEFINE N5YRDPR:
EXP(-3.8897+.0140*AJCCAGEM+.2844*AJCCSEX+.1840*AJCCSITM+.7126*AJCCTHKM+
.1785*AJCCMITM+.6932*AJCCULCM)/[1+
EXP(-3.8897+.0140*AJCCAGEM+.2844*AJCCSEX+.1840*AJCCSITM+.7126*AJCCTHKM+
.1785*AJCCMITM+.6932*AJCCULCM)]
```

The N5YRDPR attribute assigns an individual probability of experiencing death
due to metastatic melanoma within five years of diagnosis to each of the 1,222
patients based on the above six AJCC traditional prognostic factors when each
missing observation is replaced by the mean of the nonmissing observations for
that prognostic factor. These 1,222 individual probabilities were then
subjected to a ROC/AUC analysis.

The area under the complete ROC curve was estimated to be 0.7624.

Comparison of these results with those displayed in section 3.2 shows few
striking changes due to treating missing observations in the commonly practiced
factor-centered manner, except for an increase in effective sample size from
849 to 1,222 and the consequent improvement in the likelihood ratio chi-square
statistic. There was also a slight deterioration in the goodness of statistical
fit with the logistic regression model and a small increase in AUC of 0.0031,
from 0.7593 to 0.7624. The improved AUC of 0.7624 will serve as our revised
factor-centered base case level for all subsequent comparisons.

The next revised analysis replicated the previous practice-centered base case
logistic regression. The same dummy variables were used to represent the AJCC
staging classification scheme. This time, however, patients with missing
observations of initial AJCC stage were assigned five-year disease-specific
death probabilities according to the incidence of that focal event among all
patients with such missing observations in their risk subgroup.

RESULTS OF LOGISTIC REGRESSION ANALYSIS (LINEAR MODEL)

The dependent variable is a binary-coded numeric variable whose values are
either 0 or 1. It is embodied in the first expression (parameter) of the LOGREG
command, which is just the attribute DSSDUMMY.

The independent variable EXPRESSION2 is 1 IF FIRSTAGE="1a" ELSE 0.
The independent variable EXPRESSION3 is 1 IF FIRSTAGE="1b" ELSE 0.
The independent variable EXPRESSION4 is 1 IF FIRSTAGE="2a" ELSE 0.
The independent variable EXPRESSION5 is 1 IF FIRSTAGE="2b" ELSE 0.
The independent variable EXPRESSION6 is 1 IF FIRSTAGE="2c" ELSE 0.
The independent variable EXPRESSION7 is 1 IF FIRSTAGE="3a" ELSE 0.
The independent variable EXPRESSION8 is 1 IF FIRSTAGE="3b" ELSE 0.
The independent variable EXPRESSION9 is 1 IF FIRSTAGE="3c" ELSE 0.

Likelihood ratio chi-square statistic: 184.002, two-tail p value: .0000 (based
on 8 degrees of freedom and 1222 complete observations).

INDEPENDENT VARIABLE	REGRESSION COEFFICIENT	STANDARD DEVIATION	CHI-SQUARE (DF = 1)	2-TAIL P VALUE	ODDS RATIO MULTIPLIER
intercept	−1.0609	.1579	45.1466	.0000	.3462
EXPRESSION2	−1.8569	.5371	11.9541	.0005	.1562
EXPRESSION3	−1.7658	.2894	37.2192	.0000	.1711
EXPRESSION4	−.5833	.3084	3.5765	.0586	.5581
EXPRESSION5	−.1248	.2903	.1847	.6674	.8827
EXPRESSION6	.5754	.3037	3.5891	.0582	1.7778
EXPRESSION7	−.3501	.3864	.8209	.3649	.7046
EXPRESSION8	.3018	.2414	1.5621	.2114	1.3522
EXPRESSION9	1.2477	.2236	31.1431	.0000	3.4825

[Technical note: Eight zero-one dummy variables served as the independent
variables. Patients whose initial AJCC stage could not be determined were
assigned zero values on all eight dummy variables. Also, all patients initially
diagnosed in stage 4 died within five years of metastatic melanoma. They were
likewise assigned zero values on all eight dummy variables.]

RESULTS OF LOGISTIC REGRESSION ANALYSIS (LINEAR MODEL)

The dependent variable is a binary-coded numeric variable whose values are
either 0 or 1. It is embodied in the first expression (parameter) of the LOGREG
command, which is just the attribute DSSDUMMY.

The independent variable EXPRESSION2 is 1 IF RISKLEVL=MEDRISK ELSE 0.
The independent variable EXPRESSION3 is 1 IF RISKLEVL=HIGHRISK ELSE 0.

Likelihood ratio chi-square statistic: 46.142, two-tail p value: .0000 (based
on 2 degrees of freedom and 203 complete observations).

INDEPENDENT VARIABLE	REGRESSION COEFFICIENT	STANDARD DEVIATION	CHI-SQUARE (DF = 1)	2-TAIL P VALUE	ODDS RATIO MULTIPLIER
intercept	-2.9755	.4585	42.1199	.0000	.0510
EXPRESSION2	2.1954	.5855	14.0605	.0002	8.9833
EXPRESSION3	2.8832	.5214	30.5752	.0000	17.8706

[Technical note: Two zero-one dummy variables served as the independent
variables. Patients in the low-risk subgroup were assigned zero values on both
dummy variables. This dummy-variable logistic regression was performed only on
the 203 patients whose initial AJCC stage could not be determined.]

DEFINE F5YRDPR:
EXP(-1.0609-1.8569)/[1+EXP(-1.0609-1.8569)] IF FIRSTAGE="1a" ELSE
EXP(-1.0609-1.7658)/[1+EXP(-1.0609-1.7658)] IF FIRSTAGE="1b" ELSE
EXP(-1.0609-.5833)/[1+EXP(-1.0609-.5833)] IF FIRSTAGE="2a" ELSE
EXP(-1.0609-.1248)/[1+EXP(-1.0609-.1248)] IF FIRSTAGE="2b" ELSE
EXP(-1.0609+.5754)/[1+EXP(-1.0609+.5754)] IF FIRSTAGE="2c" ELSE
EXP(-1.0609-.3501)/[1+EXP(-1.0609-.3501)] IF FIRSTAGE="3a" ELSE
EXP(-1.0609+.3018)/[1+EXP(-1.0609+.3018)] IF FIRSTAGE="3b" ELSE
EXP(-1.0609+1.2477)/[1+EXP(-1.0609+1.2477)] IF FIRSTAGE="3c" ELSE
1.0000 IF FIRSTAGE="4" ELSE
EXP(-2.9755)/[1+EXP(-2.9755)] IF RISKLEVL=LOWRISK ELSE
EXP(-2.9755+2.1954)/[1+EXP(-2.9755+2.1954)] IF RISKLEVL=MEDRISK ELSE
EXP(-2.9755+2.8832)/[1+EXP(-2.9755+2.8832)] IF RISKLEVL=HIGHRISK

The F5YRDPR attribute assigns an individual probability of experiencing death
due to metastatic melanoma within five years of diagnosis to each of the 1,222
patients based solely on AJCC stage at diagnosis as a classificatory
(dummy-variable) input to logistic regression. When initial AJCC stage could
not be determined, patients were assigned five-year disease-specific death
probabilities according to the incidence of that focal event among all patients
with such missing observations in their risk subgroup. These 1,222 individual
probabilities were then subjected to a ROC/AUC analysis.

The area under the complete ROC curve was estimated to be 0.7867.

Substituting the initial AJCC staging classification for the AJCC six
traditional factors increased the AUC by 0.0243, from 0.7624 to 0.7867. It also
produced an index of error reduction = 0.3257 compared to the revised
factor-centered base case analysis. A Wilcoxon test was performed on the 1,222
matched pairs of probabilistic prediction errors, showing a normalized Z
statistic = 6.93, with a two-tail p value < 0.00005.

Each prognostic factor's optimal scale partitioning and numeric rescaling is
embodied in its univariate impact-reflecting index (UIRI) produced by the Scale
Partitioning and Spacing Algorithm (SPSA). The six UIRI indexes were
substituted for their corresponding six AJCC traditional prognostic factors,
and the following logistic regression analysis was performed.

RESULTS OF LOGISTIC REGRESSION ANALYSIS (LINEAR MODEL)

The dependent variable is a binary-coded numeric variable whose values are either 0 or 1. It is embodied in the first expression (parameter) of the LOGREG command, which is just the attribute DSSDUMMY.

The independent variable AGEAUIRI is just the attribute AGEAUIRI.
The independent variable SEXAUIRI is just the attribute SEXAUIRI.
The independent variable SITAUIRI is just the attribute SITAUIRI.
The independent variable THKAUIRI is just the attribute THKAUIRI.
The independent variable MITAUIRI is just the attribute MITAUIRI.
The independent variable ULCAUIRI is just the attribute ULCAUIRI.

Likelihood ratio chi-square statistic: 234.144, two-tail p value: .0000 (based on 6 degrees of freedom and 1222 complete observations).

INDEPENDENT VARIABLE	REGRESSION COEFFICIENT	STANDARD DEVIATION	CHI-SQUARE (DF = 1)	2-TAIL P VALUE	ODDS RATIO MULTIPLIER
intercept	-6.6409	1.4016	22.4502	.0000	.0013
AGEAUIRI	2.9775	1.2859	5.3618	.0206	19.6390
SEXAUIRI	4.5658	2.4037	3.6080	.0575	96.1365
SITAUIRI	6.0588	5.9012	1.0542	.3046	427.8796
THKAUIRI	4.3905	.5496	63.8193	.0000	80.6777
MITAUIRI	2.5008	.5942	17.7097	.0000	12.1917
ULCAUIRI	1.7860	.6851	6.7971	.0091	5.9658

GOODNESS OF STATISTICAL FIT OF LOGISTIC REGRESSION MODEL

Pearson chi-square fit statistic (based on 897 degrees of freedom): 870.201, p value: .7342.

Deviance chi-square fit statistic (based on 897 degrees of freedom): 885.783, p value: .6002.

DEFINE A5YRDPR:
EXP(-6.6409+2.9775*AGEAUIRI+4.5658*SEXAUIRI+6.0588*SITAUIRI+4.3905*THKAUIRI+
2.5008*MITAUIRI+1.7860*ULCAUIRI)/[1+
EXP(-6.6409+2.9775*AGEAUIRI+4.5658*SEXAUIRI+6.0588*SITAUIRI+4.3905*THKAUIRI+
2.5008*MITAUIRI+1.7860*ULCAUIRI)]

The A5YRDPR attribute assigns an individual probability of experiencing death due to metastatic melanoma within five years of diagnosis to each of the 1,222 patients based on the above six AJCC traditional prognostic factors converted by SPSA to corresponding UIRI values, but without any reference to AJCC stage at diagnosis. These 1,222 individual probabilities were then subjected to a ROC/AUC analysis.

The area under the complete ROC curve was estimated to be 0.7886.

Converting the six AJCC traditional prognostic factors to corresponding UIRI values (utilizing the SPSA technique for substituting missing observation values described in section 2.7) increased AUC by 0.0262, from 0.7624 to 0.7886, compared to the revised factor-centered base case. The index of error reduction was 0.2668. A Wilcoxon test performed on the 1,222 matched pairs of probabilistic prediction errors generated a normalized Z statistic = 7.86, with a two-tail p value < 0.00005. It also produced a noticeably better statistical fit with the logistic regression model. Compared to the revised practice-centered base case, however, the improvement in AUC was smaller and statistically insignificant (0.0019, from 0.7867 to 0.7886).

When a prognostic factor is dichotomous, substituting corresponding UIRI values as an independent variable input to logistic regression produces no predictive improvement. Patient sex, anatomical location of primary tumor, and ulceration are treated by the AJCC as possessing only two possible data values each. Therefore, excluding the way SPSA handles missing observations, the predictive improvement produced by defining the A5YRDPR attribute is entirely attributable to patient age, primary tumor thickness, and mitotic rate. Figures 2, 3, and 4 show substitute UIRI scattergrams for these three traditional prognostic factors.

Clark level of primary tumor invasion was once included in the list of traditional AJCC prognostic factors for melanoma patients. It is still involved in defining AJCC stage. Figure 5 shows the substitute UIRI scattergram for Clark level.

Comparison of Figures 2, 3, 4, and 5 shows how diverse the impact of even traditional prognostic factors can be. The diversity depicted here is in the shapes of the relationships linking each separate factor to MM death within five years of diagnosis. SPSA detects such diversity, and PCM exploits it to improve predictive accuracy.

The last analysis of traditional prognostic factors was designed to assess the incremental improvement in predictive accuracy realizable from stratifying patients into low-risk, medium-risk, and high-risk subgroups—given that the six UIRI indexes had been substituted for their corresponding six AJCC traditional factors as independent variable inputs to logistic regression. Three separate logistic regressions were executed, one on each risk subgroup. This required executing SPSA three times to produce a UIRI value for each of the six AJCC traditional prognostic factors, separately, for each risk subgroup.

All three regression analyses generated highly significant likelihood ratio chi-square statistics. The three separate regression outputs are not shown below, nor is the expression used to merge the three sets of results into the combined attribute, S5YRDPR. The same outputs and procedures were illustrated in the previous analysis of 849 patients with no missing observations. The 1,222 individual probabilities calculated for S5YRDPR (which accounts for missing observations) were then subjected to a ROC/AUC analysis.

The area under the complete ROC curve was estimated to be 0.8208.

Stratifying patients into low-risk, medium-risk, and high-risk subgroups and converting traditional prognostic factors to corresponding UIRI values improved predictive accuracy relative to all three previous revised analyses, while still preserving a more or less reasonable goodness of statistical fit of the logistic regression model. This combined procedure increased the AUC by 0.0322, from 0.7886 to 0.8208, compared to simply converting traditional prognostic factors to corresponding UIRI values, which generated the most accurate of the three previous predictions. It also generated an index of error reduction = 0.3993. A Wilcoxon test was performed on the 1,222 matched pairs of probabilistic prediction errors, producing a normalized Z statistic = 10.69, with a two-tail p value < 0.00005.

Figure 2

Scattergram of UIRI for Age at Initial Diagnosis

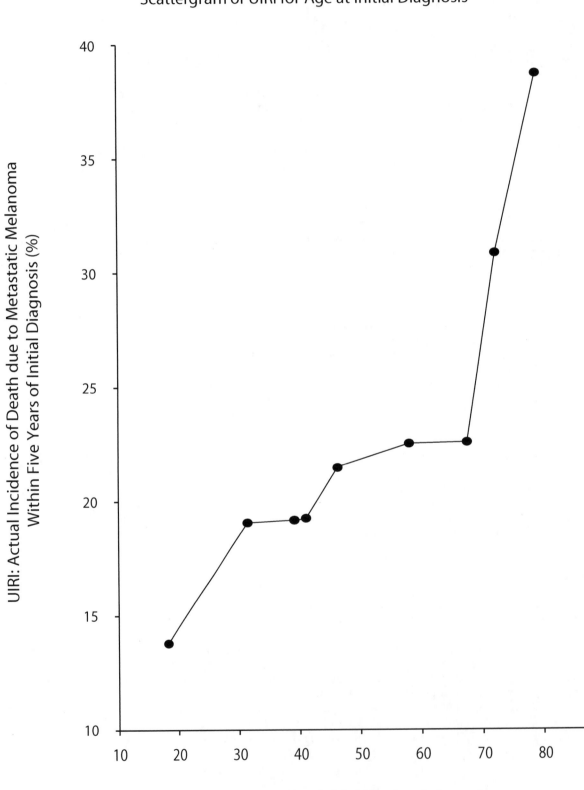

Mean Age at Initial Diagnosis (years)

Figure 3

Scattergram of UIRI for Thickness of Primary Tumor

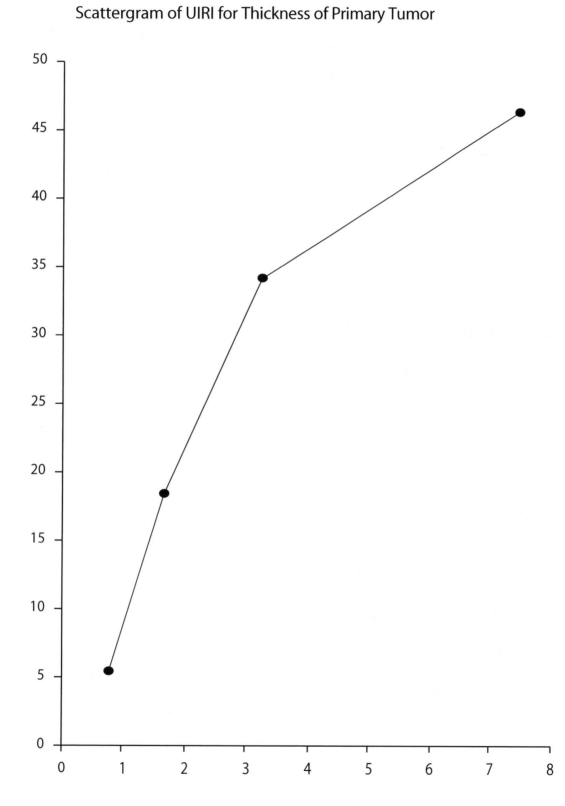

Figure 4

Scattergram of UIRI for Mitotic Rate of Primary Tumor

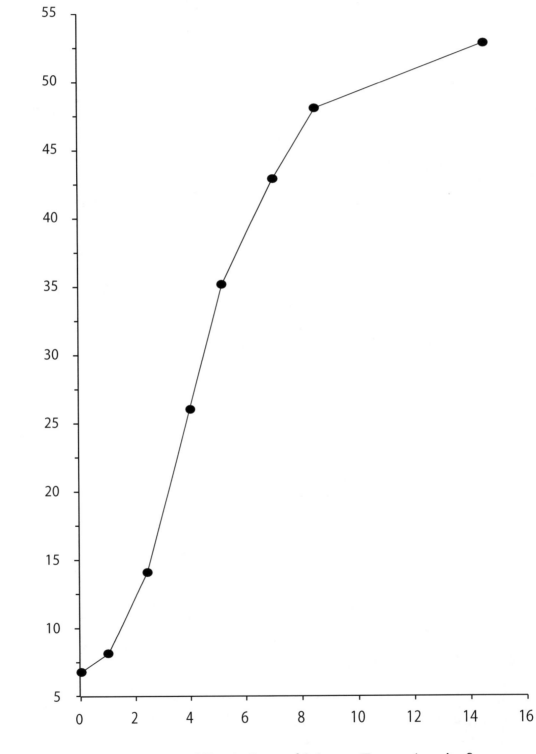

Mean Mitotic Rate of Primary Tumor (per hpf)

Figure 5

Scattergram of UIRI for Clark Level of Primary Tumor

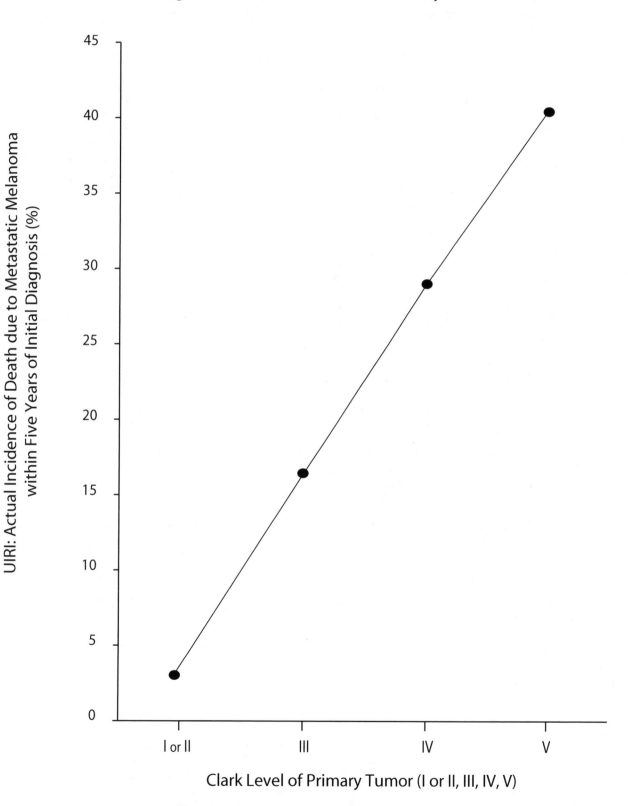

Some additional comparisons are appropriate, as follows.

1. Recall that the N5YRDPR attribute assigned an individual probability of experiencing death due to metastatic melanoma within five years of diagnosis to each of the 1,222 patients based on a standard, factor-centered logistic regression analysis of the six AJCC traditional prognostic factors. When preparing factor inputs to the logistic regression, each missing observation was replaced by the mean of the nonmissing observations of that prognostic factor.

2. Recall also that the F5YRDPR attribute based its individual probabilities of experiencing death due to metastatic melanoma solely on AJCC stage at diagnosis as a classificatory (dummy-variable) input to logistic regression. When initial AJCC stage could not be determined, patients were assigned five-year disease-specific death probabilities according to the incidence of that focal event among all patients with such missing observations in their risk subgroup.

3. The attribute just calculated, S5YRDPR, first stratified patients by risk subgroup and then substituted corresponding UIRI values for the six AJCC traditional prognostic factors (separately by risk subgroup) to produce its five-year individual death probabilities.

4. S5YRDPR embodies our proposed PCM approach when applied just to the six AJCC traditional prognostic factors. Now we must demonstrate that combining the predictive information contained in the N5YRDPR attribute with the (partially overlapping) information contained in the F5YRDPR attribute in the PCM manner produces more accurate individually tailored five-year disease-specific death predictions than if the same information were combined via standard logistic regression.

5. In section 3.1, the six AJCC traditional factors and the equivalent of F5YRDPR (both without missing observations) served as inputs to a standard logistic regression analysis. This time, N5YRDPR was substituted for the six AJCC traditional factors. When combined with F5YRDPR as a second independent variable, the resulting logistic regression accounted for all missing data. Its output was converted, as usual, to individual MM death probabilities and labeled NF5YRDPR.

6. A ROC analysis of NF5YRDPR produced an AUC of 0.7994. This constituted an AUC increase of 0.0370 compared to N5YRDPR, with a corresponding index of error reduction = 0.3519. The error reduction was significant, with a two-tail $p < 0.00005$ via a Wilcoxon test that generated a normalized Z statistic = 9.29.

7. The ROC analysis of NF5YRDPR produced an AUC increase of 0.0127 compared to F5YRDPR. Interestingly, the corresponding error reduction was quite small and not statistically significant according to the Wilcoxon test. Once a patient's initial stage at diagnosis has been ascertained, further information concerning the traditional six AJCC factors analyzed in the traditional manner seems to add insignificant predictive power.

8. In stark contrast, however, our PCM approach (S5YRDPR) produced an AUC of 0.8208. This constituted an AUC increase of 0.0214 compared to NF5YRDPR, with a corresponding index of error reduction = 0.2979. The error reduction was significant, with a two-tail $p < 0.00005$ via a Wilcoxon test that generated a normalized Z statistic = 6.53.

All of these results show that our PCM approach produced significantly more accurate individual probabilistic predictions (in terms of both AUC values and probabilistic prediction errors) than any of the other prognostic methodologies, including the commonly practiced procedure of basing predictions solely on initial AJCC staging classification. Also, the manner in which SPSA handles missing observations seemed to enhance rather than to dilute the accuracy improvement realized in the absence of missing observations.

3.4   Adding Nontraditional Prognostic Factors to the Analysis

Two groups of nontraditional prognostic factors were then added to the six
traditional AJCC factors in predicting MM death within five years for the 1,222
melanoma patients.

The first nontraditional group included nine histological factors, all of which
were ascertainable at the time of initial diagnosis:

1. primary tumor's histological subtype (see appendix B for a detailed
   list of subtypes);
2. Clark level of primary tumor invasion—risk increases with greater
   invasion;
3. level of primary tumor-infiltrating lymphocytes (TIL level)—risk
   decreases with higher level;
4. presence or absence of microsatellites—risk increases when present;
5. vascular involvement (impending or actual vascular invasion)—risk
   increases with greater involvement;
6. degree of primary tumor vascularity (angiogenesis)—risk increases with
   greater degree of vascularization;
7. degree of primary tumor regression—risk increases with higher degree
   of regression;
8. number of positive lymph nodes—risk increases with number of positive
   nodes detected at diagnosis; and
9. patient's within-risk-subgroup AJCC stage—risk increases with later
   stages.

The second nontraditional group included nine molecular factors, which were
also ascertainable at the time of initial diagnosis. These factors were
detected expressions of the following nine genes within the primary tumor,
where degree of expression was uniformly assessed according to the
pathologist's four-point scale (absent, slight, moderate, or intense staining
intensity derived from immunohistochemical protein analysis), and where higher
degrees of gene expression uniformly indicated higher risk:

1. NCOA3;
2. SPP1 (also referred to as osteopontin);
3. RGS1;
4. WNT2;
5. FN1;
6. ARPC2;
7. PHIP;
8. POU5; and
9. P65 subunit of NF-kB.

Unfortunately, usable tissue was available for only 375 of the 1,222 melanoma
patients. For this second nontraditional factor group, therefore, SPSA's
ability to deal with missing observations was seriously tested.

One reason why PCM divides prognostic factors into separate groups is to
accommodate current practice. A complete set of observations is almost never
collected. For most patients, complete data are recorded only on traditional
factors. This suggests constructing separate predictive algorithms in a
cumulative manner for patients with increasing numbers of recorded factors. The
procedure is described on the next page.

Based on the prediction improvements already achieved for the six AJCC traditional prognostic factors, the nine factors in the first nontraditional group were converted by SPSA to corresponding UIRI values exactly as previously described. The composite collection of fifteen converted UIRI factors was then subjected to three separate logistic regression analyses, one for each of the three risk subgroups of melanoma patients. The results of the three separate logistic regressions were merged into a composite attribute called G15YRDPR, also in the same manner as previously described. The 1,222 individual probabilities calculated for G15YRDPR (which accounts for missing observations of both the six traditional and the nine nontraditional factors in the first group) were then subjected to a ROC/AUC analysis.

The area under the complete ROC curve was estimated to be 0.8561.

Adding the new histological information encapsulated within the nine factors in the first nontraditional group to the six traditional AJCC factors increased the AUC by 0.0353, from 0.8208 achieved by S5YRDPR to 0.8561 achieved by G15YRDPR, and increased to a highly respectable level the goodness of statistical fit of the logistic regression model. It also produced an index of error reduction = 0.2422. A Wilcoxon test was performed on these 1,222 matched pairs of probabilistic prediction errors, resulting in a normalized Z statistic = 8.66, with a two-tail p value < 0.00005.

The nine molecular factors in the second nontraditional group were then converted by SPSA to corresponding UIRI values exactly as previously described, and the composite collection of twenty-four converted UIRI factors was then subjected to three separate logistic regression analyses, one for each of the three risk subgroups of melanoma patients. The results of the three separate logistic regressions were merged into a composite attribute called G25YRDPR, also in the same manner as previously described. The 1,222 individual probabilities calculated for G25YRDPR (which accounts for missing observations of the six traditional factors, the nine histological factors in the first nontraditional group, and the nine molecular factors in the second nontraditional group) were then subjected to a ROC/AUC analysis.

The area under the complete ROC curve was estimated to be 0.8656.

Adding the new molecular information encapsulated within the nine factors in the second nontraditional group to the six traditional AJCC factors and the nine histological factors in the first nontraditional group increased the AUC by 0.0095, from 0.8561 achieved by G15YRDPR to 0.8656 achieved by G25YRDPR, and increased the goodness of statistical fit of the logistic regression model to a still higher level. This occurred despite the large number of missing observations among the nine molecular factors. It also produced an index of error reduction = 0.2193. A Wilcoxon test was performed on these 1,222 matched pairs of probabilistic prediction errors, resulting in a normalized Z statistic = 6.74, with a two-tail p value < 0.00005.

3.5   Summary of Melanoma Results

The addition of eighteen nontraditional prognostic factors to six traditional factors, with all twenty-four factors analyzed according to our proposed patient-centered methodology, produced the following improvements in predictive accuracy.

1. Compared to the traditional factor-centered base case, AUC increased by 10.32 percentage points, from 76.24 percent to 86.56 percent. The

maximum achievable percentage of correct predictions increased by 4.74 points, from 78.81 percent to 83.55 percent.

2. Compared to the practice-centered base case, AUC increased by 7.89 percentage points, from 78.67 percent to 86.56 percent. The maximum achievable percentage of correct predictions increased by 4.74 points, from 78.81 percent to 83.55 percent.

3. All of these increases compare quite favorably with the meager two-percentage-point AUC improvement reported by Dr. Ware in 2006, where statistically significant nontraditional prognostic factors were added to traditional factors in a standard factor-centered analysis—but without the benefit of PCM.

4. As measured by the index of error reduction and the Wilcoxon matched-pairs, signed-ranks tests, these improvements were highly significant, all showing two-tail p values < 0.00005.

Shown below are summary statistics for the individual patient probabilities of experiencing death due to metastatic melanoma within five years of diagnosis produced by the six logistic regression analyses (N5YRDPR, F5YRDPR, A5YRDPR, S5YRDPR, G15YRDPR, and G25YRDPR).

Notice that the mean probabilities are all identical and equal to the incidence of death due to metastatic melanoma among these 1,222 patients. This pleasant feature of logistic regression analysis has already been alluded to.

Notice also the differences in the minimum-to-maximum ranges and the standard deviations of these individual probabilities. Not only does G25YRDPR produce the most accurate probabilistic predictions (as just shown in terms of AUC, maximum achievable percentage of correct predictions, and probabilistic prediction error), it also tends to "spread out" its probabilistic predictions more widely than the other five probabilistic logistic regression outputs. Finer discrimination is achieved in combination with greater accuracy, not at the expense of greater accuracy.

SUMMARY STATISTICS	ATTRIBUTE DSSDUMMY	
n DEFINED	1222	
MINIMUM	0	DSSDUMMY = 0 means survival for more than five years.
MEDIAN	0	
MAXIMUM	1	DSSDUMMY = 1 means MM death within five years.
MEAN	.2300	
STD. DEV.	.4208	

SUMMARY STATISTICS	ATTRIBUTE N5YRDPR	ATTRIBUTE F5YRDPR	ATTRIBUTE A5YRDPR	ATTRIBUTE S5YRDPR	ATTRIBUTE G15YRDPR	ATTRIBUTE G25YRDPR
n DEFINED	1222	1222	1222	1222	1222	1222
MINIMUM	.0411	.0485	.0355	.0113	.0018	.0016
MEDIAN	.1501	.1961	.1532	.1573	.1309	.1202
MAXIMUM	.6018	1.0000	.8285	.7480	.9301	.9810
MEAN	.2300	.2300	.2300	.2300	.2300	.2300
STD. DEV.	.1683	.1881	.1863	.2070	.2333	.2408

G25YRDPR was the most accurate predictor in all of the above senses. Investigation of its scale characteristics throughout its complete logical range from zero to one will reveal other senses in which its probabilistic predictions were also remarkably reliable.

The United States Weather Bureau faces a similar task in assessing its probabilistic predictions for accuracy and reliability. The bureau makes daily forecasts covering all kinds of weather. Imagine that the chance of rain for a given day at some location is announced to be a number between 20 and 30 percent. As more and more forecasts are made, the mean of all daily probabilistic predictions announcing the chance of rain to fall between 20 and 30 percent should gradually converge toward the actual incidence of rain at that same location during those same days. Also, the actual incidence should fall within the 20 to 30 percent interval. In like manner, mean probabilistic predictions in all other intervals throughout the entire range of forecasts should gradually converge toward their corresponding actual incidences, and the incidences eventually realized should always fall within their respective intervals.

The 1,222 G25YRDPR individually tailored probabilities were first ranked and divided into quartiles. The mean of the probabilities in each quartile was then compared with the actual incidence of MM death within five years of diagnosis among the patients in that quartile.

These two numbers should be about the same in each quartile. The maximum absolute difference was 1.95 percentage points. The mean absolute difference was 0.98 percentage points. Furthermore, there was no discernible pattern or trend in the succession of quartile probabilities and incidences.

When there are only a few distinctly different probability values in a data set, partitioning the scale into a small number of subscales, such as quartiles, may be an appropriate procedure. There were 1,131 distinctly different values of G25YRDPR. Consequently, we can investigate its scale characteristics much more thoroughly.

The SPSA algorithm was executed to partition the scale of G25YRDPR into as many subscales as possible, as long as each subscale encompassed MM death probabilities for at least 25 patients. Seventeen separate subscales were produced. They are shown below as SPSA's printed output. The corresponding actual incidence of MM death within five years of diagnosis is shown as a fraction for each subscale.

```
4/277 IF G25YRDPR<.0305 ELSE
1/50 IF G25YRDPR>=.0305 AND G25YRDPR<.0391 ELSE
1/31 IF G25YRDPR>=.0391 AND G25YRDPR<.0448 ELSE
1/28 IF G25YRDPR>=.0448 AND G25YRDPR<.0508 ELSE
2/53 IF G25YRDPR>=.0508 AND G25YRDPR<.0626 ELSE
2/50 IF G25YRDPR>=.0626 AND G25YRDPR<.0767 ELSE
7/99 IF G25YRDPR>=.0767 AND G25YRDPR<.1129 ELSE
6/42 IF G25YRDPR>=.1129 AND G25YRDPR<.1314 ELSE
22/129 IF G25YRDPR>=.1314 AND G25YRDPR<.2107 ELSE
10/41 IF G25YRDPR>=.2107 AND G25YRDPR<.2453 ELSE
18/67 IF G25YRDPR>=.2453 AND G25YRDPR<.3235 ELSE
16/48 IF G25YRDPR>=.3235 AND G25YRDPR<.3847 ELSE
30/65 IF G25YRDPR>=.3847 AND G25YRDPR<.4832 ELSE
22/41 IF G25YRDPR>=.4832 AND G25YRDPR<.528 ELSE
57/86 IF G25YRDPR>=.528 AND G25YRDPR<.6483 ELSE
34/51 IF G25YRDPR>=.6483 AND G25YRDPR<.723 ELSE
48/64 IF G25YRDPR>=.723
```

The table on the following page was then constructed. Prediction errors were calculated for each successive subscale as the mean of the G25YRDPR values falling within that subscale subtracted from the actual incidence of MM death within five years among the patients possessing those values of G25YRDPR.

SUBSCALE	LOWER AND UPPER SUBSCALE BOUNDS		SUBSCALE MEAN	ACTUAL INCIDENCE	PREDICTION ERROR
1	.0000 to	.0305	.0148	.0144	-.0004
2	.0305 to	.0391	.0340	.0200	-.0140
3	.0391 to	.0448	.0424	.0323	-.0101
4	.0448 to	.0508	.0468	.0357	-.0111
5	.0508 to	.0626	.0563	.0377	-.0186
6	.0626 to	.0767	.0698	.0400	-.0298
7	.0767 to	.1129	.0965	.0707	-.0258
8	.1129 to	.1314	.1204	.1429	.0225
9	.1314 to	.2107	.1691	.1705	.0014
10	.2107 to	.2453	.2284	.2439	.0155
11	.2453 to	.3235	.2849	.2687	-.0162
12	.3235 to	.3847	.3506	.3333	-.0173
13	.3847 to	.4832	.4360	.4615	.0255
14	.4832 to	.5280	.5069	.5366	.0297
15	.5280 to	.6483	.5793	.6628	.0835
16	.6483 to	.7230	.6842	.6667	-.0175
17	.7230 to	1.0000	.7902	.7500	-.0402

Since the number of subscales expanded from four (quartiles) to seventeen, subscales contained fewer patient probabilities (between 28 and 277 each). Therefore, the convergence process was rendered less complete. The maximum absolute difference between the seventeen subscale means and their corresponding actual incidences was 8.35 percentage points. The mean absolute difference was 2.23 percentage points.

Taking algebraic signs into account, the mean prediction error should be very close to zero. It was -0.13 percentage points. Both a one-sample T test and a corresponding Wilcoxon test suggested that the population of prediction errors from which this sample of seventeen was drawn differed insignificantly from one with a mean and a median of zero.

When successive subscale means were plotted along the horizontal X-axis and the corresponding actual incidences were plotted along the vertical Y-axis of a graph, all seventeen points fell close to the straight line through the origin that makes a 45-degree angle with each axis. This line assumes that every actual incidence exactly equals its corresponding subscale mean. Prediction errors are vertical deviations from the line. The R squared value associated with this line, interpreted as a simple linear regression equation, was 0.9868 (equivalent to a 0.9934 linear correlation coefficient).

Inspection of the sequence of prediction errors revealed six positive and eleven negative errors, with relatively large and relatively small prediction errors clustered neither at the extremes of the probability scale nor in its interior. These results were consistent with a random pattern of errors. There was, however, a noticeable tendency for the absolute size of prediction errors to rise with larger probability numbers in the scale.

Based on these observations, it seems appropriate to conclude that individually tailored G25YRDPR probabilities provide quite accurate predictions of whether or not a melanoma patient will experience MM death within five years of initial diagnosis—especially at low and intermediate probability levels. Figure 6 provides visual evidence of their predictive accuracy.

Figure 6

Scattergram of Predictive Accuracy of
G25YRDPR Composite Probability

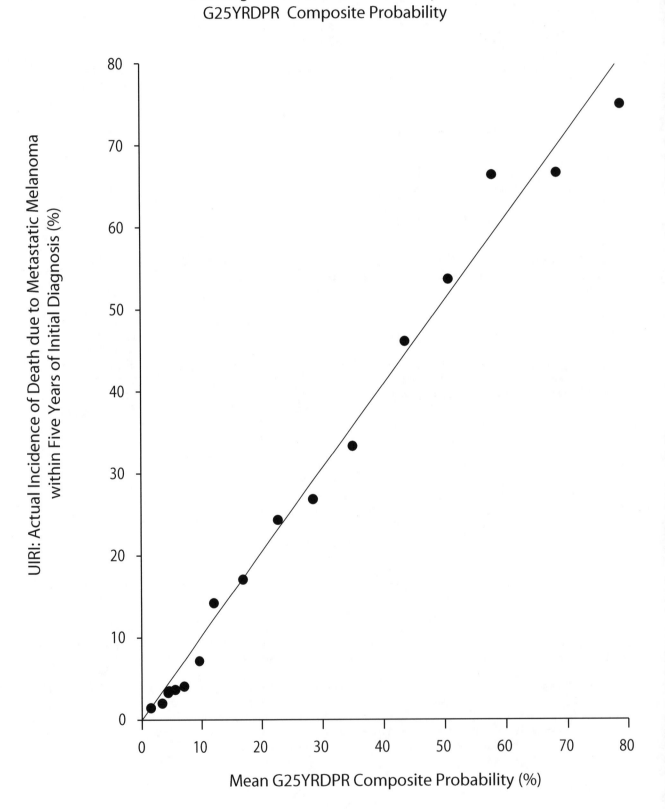

UIRI: Actual Incidence of Death due to Metastatic Melanoma within Five Years of Initial Diagnosis (%)

Mean G25YRDPR Composite Probability (%)

Figure 7 displays the four most salient ROC plots resulting from the melanoma analysis:

1. the ROC plot based on the factor-centered base case analysis of the six AJCC traditional prognostic factors, analyzed in the usual, factor-centered manner (N5YRDPR);
2. the ROC plot based on the practice-centered base case analysis—a dummy-variable logistic regression of initial AJCC stage (F5YRDPR);
3. the ROC plot based on the same six AJCC traditional prognostic factors, but now analyzed via our proposed patient-centered methodology, which uses AJCC stage at diagnosis as a stratifying variable for logistic regression and uniformly substitutes UIRI values for all prognostic factors (S5YRDPR); and
4. the ROC plot based on adding eighteen nontraditional factors to the same six AJCC traditional prognostic factors, again analyzed via our proposed patient-centered methodology (G25YRDPR).

Section 2.8 described how to weight the relative predictive potency of the six AJCC traditional prognostic factors, the nine nontraditional histological factors, and the nine nontraditional molecular factors. These weights are tabled in appendix C.

The weight assigned to any factor in a risk subgroup (column of appendix C) indicates the predictive potency of that factor relative to the other factors in the same factor group. Hence, the weights add to 1.0 in each factor group and risk subgroup combination (nine combinations in all).

The explanatory notes in appendix C provide additional information on relative predictive potency weights across factor groups within separate risk subgroups. Such information would be useful in deciding exactly what additional prognostic factor information might prove most beneficial for a freshly diagnosed patient with less than complete readings on all twenty-four factors (i.e., for almost all patients).

Appendix C suggests that the relative predictive potency of separate prognostic factors varies markedly across risk subgroups. The 1,222 melanoma patients in the training sample cannot be viewed as having been drawn from a single population, homogeneous in this sense. When such heterogeneity is detected, PCM exploits it by stratifying the training sample into separate risk subgroups and repeating the analysis, separately, for each risk subgroup.

There were some commonalities across risk subgroups. For example, tumor thickness, mitotic rate, angiogenesis, FN1, and PHIP were assigned nonzero weights in all three risk subgroups. It is amazing that FN1 and PHIP made this grade. Only one quarter to one third of the 1,222 patients had recorded values of FN1 or PHIP or any of the other seven molecular factors.

Tumor thickness has long been recognized as a potent prognostic factor in melanoma. Mitotic rate has just recently been recognized by the AJCC as deserving similar attention. Vascular factors, such as angiogenesis and vascular involvement, and molecular factors, such as FN1 and PHIP, have yet to achieve similar recognition.

Figure 7

ROC Analyses

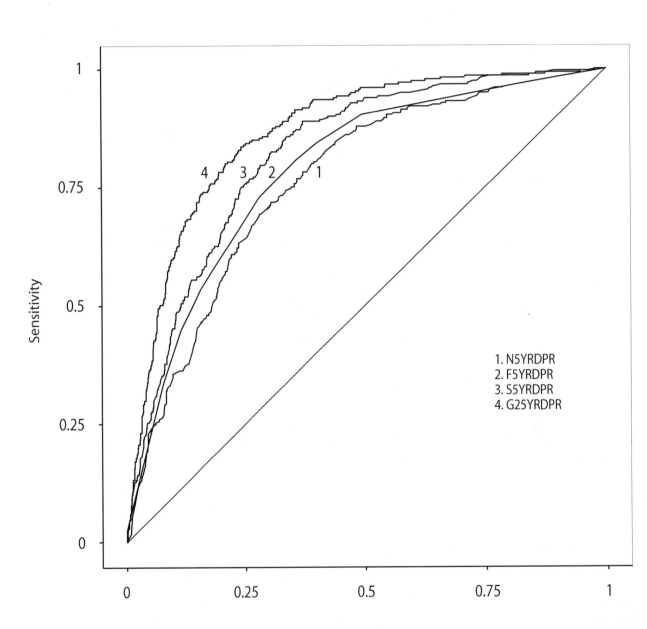

1. N5YRDPR
2. F5YRDPR
3. S5YRDPR
4. G25YRDPR

3.6 Applying Tailored Individual Probabilities to Making Therapeutic Choices

Another possible use of the individually tailored probabilities of experiencing MM death within five years of diagnosis is to aid in the selection of candidates for adjuvant therapy.

The traditional eligibility criteria for high-dose alpha-2b interferon (IFN) have included thick primary tumor (exceeding 4 millimeters) or node-positive disease or both. Using these criteria, we identified the subset of 492 patients in our training sample of 1,222 who were eligible for high-dose IFN treatment. We then ranked the 1,222 patients in decreasing order of their individually tailored probabilities of experiencing MM death within five years of diagnosis. G25YRDPR, the final and most comprehensive output of PCM, was used to make this ranking. Excluding the seven patients who were initially diagnosed in stage 4 (too late for IFN), we then identified the top-ranked subset of 492 patients in terms of their G25YRDPR probabilities.

The combined total of 619 patients included in either or both of these two subsets were assigned to the following three mutually exclusive categories:

1. category 1 containing 127 patients identified as eligible for high-dose IFN treatment by the traditional criteria, but not included within PCM's top-ranked subset of 492 patients;
2. category 2 containing 127 patients included within PCM's top-ranked subset of 492 patients, but not identified as eligible for high-dose IFN treatment by the traditional criteria; and
3. category 3 containing 365 patients both identified as eligible for high-dose IFN treatment by the traditional criteria and included within PCM's top-ranked subset of 492 patients.

Figure 8 graphs the results of a Kaplan-Meier analysis of disease-specific survival for all three categories of patients. The survival of category 2 patients appeared to be dramatically lower than the survival of category 1 patients, but indistinguishably different from the survival of category 3 patients.

Figure 9 graphs the results of a Kaplan-Meier analysis of disease-specific survival for the 127 category 1 versus the 127 category 2 patients. Their survival differed significantly (Log-rank two-tail p value < 0.0001).

Figure 10 graphs the results of a Kaplan-Meier analysis of disease-specific survival for the 127 category 2 versus the 365 category 3 patients. Their survival differed hardly at all (Log-rank two-tail p value = 0.8201).

These results suggest that the individually tailored probabilities of MM death within five years of diagnosis finally produced by PCM (values of the G25YRDPR attribute) identify high-risk patients significantly more reliably than traditional eligibility criteria for IFN treatment.

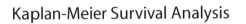

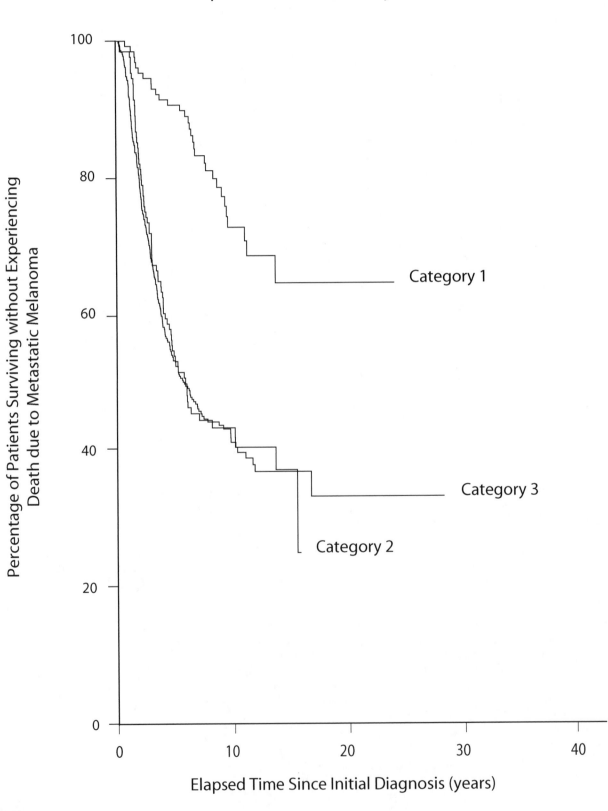

Figure 9

Kaplan-Meier Survival Analysis

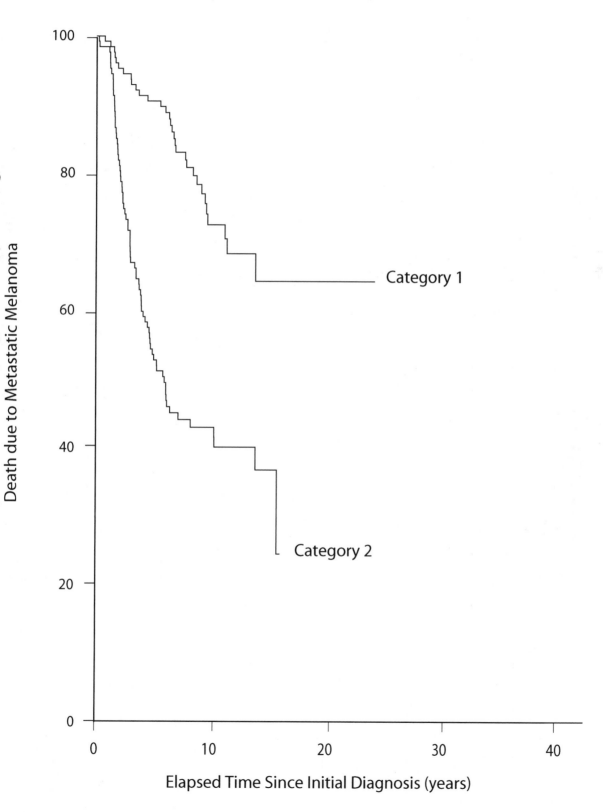

Figure 10

Kaplan-Meier Survival Analysis

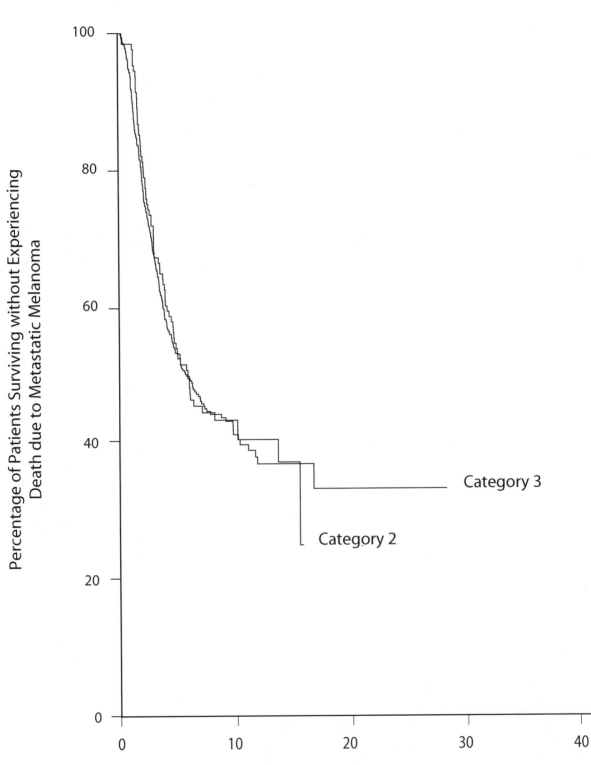

Category 3

Category 2

Percentage of Patients Surviving without Experiencing Death due to Metastatic Melanoma

Elapsed Time Since Initial Diagnosis (years)

4.0 APPLYING PCM TO 1,225 BREAST CANCER PATIENTS

As stated in section 2.1, disease-specific death within five years following initial diagnosis has been chosen as the focal event to be predicted, probabilistically, by our proposed patient-centered methodology.

A sample of 1,225 patients diagnosed with invasive breast cancer between April 1945 and December 1984 in Turku, Finland, was collected and analyzed to serve as a second illustration of PCM's ability to improve prognostic accuracy. These patients were followed up until April 1996. Median and mean follow-up periods were 8.50 and 9.97 years, respectively. Selected attributes of the Turku training sample are presented in appendix D.

All 1,225 patients either died of metastatic breast cancer within five years after diagnosis or survived for more than five years. The following table shows that 446 of the 1,225 (36.41 percent) suffered disease-specific death within five years, while the other 779 patients (63.59 percent) did not.

VALUE OF DEFINING EXPRESSION	VALUE OF ATTRIBUTE DSS5YR		
	DSS>5YRS	MBC DEATH=<5YRS	TOTAL
MBC DEATH=<5 YRS.	0	446	446
MBC DEATH>5 YRS.	224	0	224
NO MBC DEATH, F/U>5 YRS.	555	0	555
TOTAL	779	446	1225

Notes: MBC DEATH means death due to metastatic breast cancer. F/U means follow-up period in years. DSS means disease-specific survival.

4.1 Stratifying Patients into Low-Risk, Medium-Risk, and High-Risk Subgroups

The first task was to stratify the 1,225 patients into appropriate subgroups.

Among the widely understood and routinely recorded traditional prognostic factors in breast cancer, AJCC stage, tumor size, and tumor grade (which includes an assessment of mitotic count) are generally regarded as among the best single predictors of MBC death. We verified this for our 1,225-patient breast cancer training sample by selecting the subset of 677 patients with no missing observations on any traditional factors and executing the same procedures applied to the 1,222 patients in the melanoma training sample.

The more-recently discovered prognostic factors (e.g., HER2) were not regarded as candidate traditional factors. This was to ensure comparability with the melanoma analysis. Moreover, data concerning such factors were not included in the Turku data set.

The Turku data set did not record each patient's AJCC staging classification at the time of initial diagnosis. However, sufficient data on T, N, and M scale values were recorded to determine initial stage for 1,177 (96.08 percent) of them. Determinations were based on the staging criteria subsequently established by the AJCC for breast cancer.

Not surprisingly, AJCC stage at initial diagnosis also emerged as the best single predictor of five-year MBC death. When only mitotic count (but not the other components of tumor grade) was included in the multivariate logistic regression, AJCC stage, tumor size, and mitotic count were, once again, independently significant prognostic factors. Their relative predictive accuracies also fell in the same rank order as in the melanoma analysis, but between-factor differences were even more pronounced. This time, patient age at diagnosis was almost statistically significant in the multivariate analysis.

Suffice it to say that AJCC stage was an even clearer winner in breast cancer. Details of these analyses are not reported, since the procedures executed and the results achieved replicated so closely those described in section 3.1.

Also to remain comparable with the melanoma analysis, breast cancer patients were then stratified into three risk subgroups. This was accomplished by:

1. assigning all 522 patients in stages 0, 1a, 1b, and 2a to the low-risk subgroup;
2. assigning all thirty-one patients in stage 2b, 312 of 427 stage 3a patients, and twenty-seven of 103 stage 3b patients to the medium-risk subgroup;
3. assigning 115 of 427 stage 3a patients, seventy-six of 103 stage 3b patients, and all ninety-four patients in stages 3c and 4 to the high-risk subgroup; and
4. distributing the remaining patients whose AJCC stage at diagnosis could not be easily determined among the three risk subgroups according to whatever partial data were available (see next paragraph).

Detailed stratification was carried out in the following manner.

1. 286 patients were assigned to the high-risk subgroup, because:

   a. either their cancer was metastatic at diagnosis (M=1); or
   b. their cancer was not metastatic at diagnosis (M=0), but they were in at least the second nodal category (N>=2); or
   c. their cancer was not metastatic at diagnosis (M=0), but they were in the first nodal category (N=1) and in at least the third tumor category (T>=3).

2. 387 patients were assigned to the medium-risk subgroup, because:

   a. either their cancer was not metastatic at diagnosis (M=0), but they were in the first nodal category (N=1); or
   b. their cancer was not metastatic at diagnosis (M=0), and they were free of nodal involvement (N=0), but they were in at least the third tumor category (T>=3).

3. The remaining 552 patients were defined as neither high-risk nor medium-risk. By default, they were assigned to the low-risk subgroup.

This stratification produced a rank order of incidences by risk subgroup consistent with the rates of MBC death within five years of diagnosis actually experienced by patients in the Turku training sample. The following incidences were also adequate to support stable statistical estimates within subgroups.

1. 552 low-risk patients experienced an 11.41 percent incidence of MBC death.
2. 387 medium-risk patients experienced a 39.79 percent incidence of MBC death.
3. 286 high-risk patients experienced an 80.07 percent incidence of MBC death.

The dramatic between-subgroup differences in the incidence of death due to metastatic breast cancer were highly significant when assessed by a Kruskal-Wallis test corrected for tied observations (two-tail p value < 0.00005), as were the differences in DSS survival rates when assessed by Kaplan-Meier analysis (Log-rank test two-tail p value < 0.0001, Figure 11).

4.2 Analysis of Traditional Prognostic Factors without Missing Observations

Now let us adopt as a factor-centered base case five conventional (i.e., routinely recorded) prognostic factors in breast cancer analogous to the six AJCC traditional factors in melanoma. Patient sex could not be included since all breast cancer patients in the Turku training sample were female.

The five conventional base case factors were defined in a manner as similar as possible to the manner in which the AJCC defined them for melanoma. Thus, age at diagnosis was partitioned into the same conventional ten-year groupings. In the melanoma analysis this traditional factor was labeled AJCCAGE. In the breast cancer analysis the same factor is labeled CONVAGE. CONV replaced AJCC as the first four characters naming all conventional factors in breast cancer.

All five conventional factors and values of initial AJCC stage were defined at diagnosis for 677 of the 1,225 breast cancer patients. In the factor-centered approach, patients with any missing observations are typically deleted from the analysis, and there is no prior stratification by risk level. The results of a standard, factor-centered logistic regression on these five prognostic factors with no missing observations are shown directly below.

RESULTS OF LOGISTIC REGRESSION ANALYSIS (LINEAR MODEL)

The dependent variable is a binary-coded numeric variable whose values are either 0 or 1. It is embodied in the first expression (parameter) of the LOGREG command, which is just the attribute DSSDUMMY.

The independent variable CONVAGE is just the attribute CONVAGE.
The independent variable CONVSITE is just the attribute CONVSITE.
The independent variable CONVSIZE is just the attribute CONVSIZE.
The independent variable CONVMITC is just the attribute CONVMITC.
The independent variable CONVULC is just the attribute CONVULC.

Likelihood ratio chi-square statistic: 142.816, two-tail p value: .0000 (based on 5 degrees of freedom and 677 complete observations).

INDEPENDENT VARIABLE	REGRESSION COEFFICIENT	STANDARD DEVIATION	CHI-SQUARE (DF = 1)	2-TAIL P VALUE	ODDS RATIO MULTIPLIER
intercept	-4.2444	.5389	62.0230	.0000	.0143
CONVAGE	.1098	.0752	2.1339	.1441	1.1161
CONVSITE	-.0334	.2459	.0185	.8918	.9671
CONVSIZE	.5777	.0969	35.5630	.0000	1.7819
CONVMITC	1.4555	.2328	39.0917	.0000	4.2866
CONVULC	14.0274	257.8839	.0030	.9566	1236032.2350

[Technical note: CONVULC's regression coefficient is statistically unstable. All thirteen patients with ulceration died of MBC within five years of diagnosis.]

Figure 11

Kaplan-Meier Survival Analysis

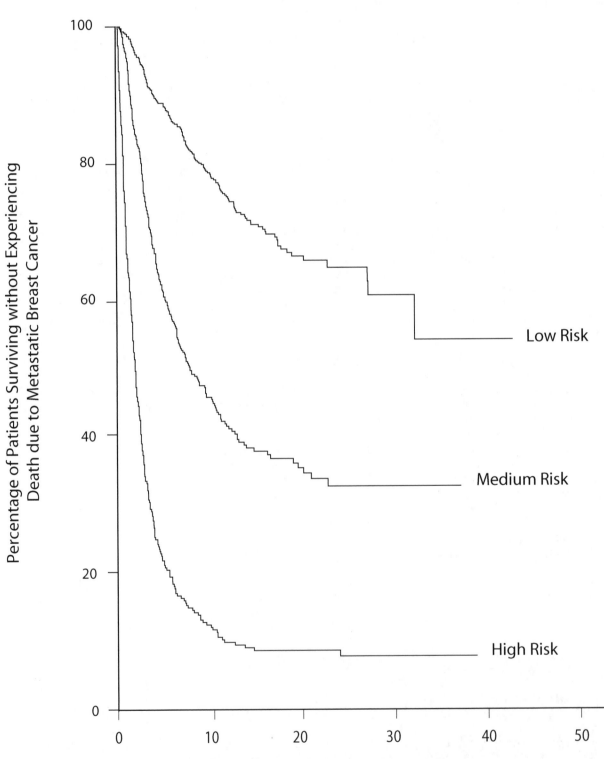

GOODNESS OF STATISTICAL FIT OF LOGISTIC REGRESSION MODEL

Pearson chi-square fit statistic (based on 88 degrees of freedom): 93.466, p value: .3250.

Deviance chi-square fit statistic (based on 88 degrees of freedom): 90.567, p value: .4045.

DEFINE CN5YRDPR:
EXP(-4.2444+.1098*CONVAGE-.0334*CONVSITE+.5777*CONVSIZE+1.4555*CONVMITC+
14.0274*CONVULC)/[1+
EXP(-4.2444+.1098*CONVAGE-.0334*CONVSITE+.5777*CONVSIZE+1.4555*CONVMITC+
14.0274*CONVULC)] IF FIRSTAGE#UNDEFS

The CN5YRDPR attribute assigns an individual probability of experiencing death due to metastatic breast cancer within five years of diagnosis to each of the 677 patients based on the above five conventional prognostic factors. These 677 individual probabilities were then subjected to a ROC/AUC analysis.

The area under the complete ROC curve was estimated to be 0.7708.

The next analysis we shall again refer to as the practice-centered base case. It recognizes that many practicing physicians in breast cancer also consider initial AJCC stage (not the five conventional breast cancer factors) as the generally accepted basis for making individual patient prognoses.

Since AJCC stage is a classification index, the practice-centered base case analysis was a logistic regression based on dummy variables. The dependent variable was MBC death within five years of diagnosis. The independent variables were zero-one dummy variables identifying, respectively, in which stage each patient was initially diagnosed. By transforming the output into probabilities, an individually tailored probabilistic prediction was made for each patient. Predictions were based on initial AJCC stage alone. There were no missing observations for the 677 patients included in this practice-centered base case analysis.

As in the melanoma analysis, the probability of MBC death within five years assigned to each of the 677 patients was its incidence among all patients classified in that patient's same initial AJCC stage. This continues to support the common practice of using incidence by stage as an individualized patient prediction when nothing else is available to make a systematic prognosis.

RESULTS OF LOGISTIC REGRESSION ANALYSIS (LINEAR MODEL)

The dependent variable is a binary-coded numeric variable whose values are either 0 or 1. It is embodied in the first expression (parameter) of the LOGREG command, which is just the attribute DSSDUMMY.

The independent variable EXPRESSION2 is 1 IF FIRSTAGE="1a" OR "1b" ELSE 0.
The independent variable EXPRESSION3 is 1 IF FIRSTAGE="2a" ELSE 0.
The independent variable EXPRESSION4 is 1 IF FIRSTAGE="2b" ELSE 0.
The independent variable EXPRESSION5 is 1 IF FIRSTAGE="3a" ELSE 0.
The independent variable EXPRESSION6 is 1 IF FIRSTAGE="3b" ELSE 0.

Likelihood ratio chi-square statistic: 190.998, two-tail p value: .0000 (based on 5 degrees of freedom and 674 complete observations).

INDEPENDENT VARIABLE	REGRESSION COEFFICIENT	STANDARD DEVIATION	CHI-SQUARE (DF = 1)	2-TAIL P VALUE	ODDS RATIO MULTIPLIER
intercept	2.1518	.4725	20.7389	.0000	8.6000
EXPRESSION2	-5.1419	.5831	77.7735	.0000	.0058
EXPRESSION3	-4.0977	.5355	58.5564	.0000	.0166
EXPRESSION4	-3.2504	.8171	15.8229	.0001	.0388
EXPRESSION5	-2.6096	.4907	28.2794	.0000	.0736
EXPRESSION6	-2.1518	.5644	14.5374	.0001	.1163

[Technical notes: Five zero-one dummy variables served as the independent variables. Patients diagnosed in either stage 1a or 1b were assigned a value of one on the first dummy variable; otherwise, zero. There were no patients without missing observations diagnosed in stage 3c. All patients diagnosed in stage 4 were assigned zero values on all five dummy variables. All three patients diagnosed in stage zero survived for more than five years. They were excluded from this practice-centered base case logistic regression analysis. Only the remaining 674 patients with no missing observations were included.]

DEFINE CF5YRDPR:
0.0000 IF FIRSTAGE="0" ELSE
EXP(2.1518-5.1419)/[1+EXP(2.1518-5.1419)] IF FIRSTAGE="1a" OR "1b" ELSE
EXP(2.1518-4.0977)/[1+EXP(2.1518-4.0977)] IF FIRSTAGE="2a" ELSE
EXP(2.1518-3.2504)/[1+EXP(2.1518-3.2504)] IF FIRSTAGE="2b" ELSE
EXP(2.1518-2.6096)/[1+EXP(2.1518-2.6096)] IF FIRSTAGE="3a" ELSE
EXP(2.1518-2.1518)/[1+EXP(2.1518-2.1518)] IF FIRSTAGE="3b" ELSE
EXP(2.1518)/[1+EXP(2.1518)] IF FIRSTAGE="4"

The CF5YRDPR attribute assigns an individual probability of experiencing death due to metastatic breast cancer within five years of diagnosis to each of the 677 patients based solely on AJCC stage at diagnosis as a classificatory (dummy-variable) input to logistic regression. These 677 individual probabilities were then subjected to a ROC/AUC analysis.

The area under the complete ROC curve was estimated to be 0.8013.

Substituting the initial AJCC staging classification for the five conventional factors increased the AUC by 0.0305, from 0.7708 to 0.8013. It also produced an index of error reduction = 0.0724 compared to the factor-centered base case analysis. A Wilcoxon matched-pairs, signed-ranks analysis was performed on the 677 matched pairs of probabilistic prediction errors, resulting in a normalized Z statistic = 3.45, with a two-tail p value = 0.0006.

Each prognostic factor's optimal scale partitioning and numeric rescaling is embodied in its univariate impact-reflecting index (UIRI) produced by the Scale Partitioning and Spacing Algorithm (SPSA). UIRI indexes were substituted for four of five corresponding conventional breast cancer prognostic factors, and the following logistic regression analysis was performed.

RESULTS OF LOGISTIC REGRESSION ANALYSIS (LINEAR MODEL)

The dependent variable is a binary-coded numeric variable whose values are either 0 or 1. It is embodied in the first expression (parameter) of the LOGREG command, which is just the attribute DSSDUMMY.

The independent variable AGECUIRI is just the attribute AGECUIRI.
The independent variable SITCUIRI is just the attribute SITCUIRI.
The independent variable SIZCUIRI is just the attribute SIZCUIRI.
The independent variable MITCUIRI is just the attribute MITCUIRI.

Likelihood ratio chi-square statistic: 159.500, two-tail p value: .0000 (based
on 4 degrees of freedom and 677 complete observations).

INDEPENDENT VARIABLE	REGRESSION COEFFICIENT	STANDARD DEVIATION	CHI-SQUARE (DF = 1)	2-TAIL P VALUE	ODDS RATIO MULTIPLIER
intercept	-4.8291	1.0855	19.7895	.0000	.0080
AGECUIRI	4.3848	1.2441	12.4211	.0004	80.2220
SITCUIRI	-.5241	3.6249	.0209	.8850	.5921
SIZCUIRI	4.4029	.5786	57.9052	.0000	81.6856
MITCUIRI	4.8313	.7481	41.7065	.0000	125.3780

[Technical note: Converting CONVULC to ULCCUIRI via SPSA was impossible because
there were only thirteen patients with ulcerated primary breast tumors—all but
one of whom were in the high-risk subgroup. The minimum scale partition size
was twenty-five patients for all conventional prognostic factors.]

GOODNESS OF STATISTICAL FIT OF LOGISTIC REGRESSION MODEL

Pearson chi-square fit statistic (based on 240 degrees of freedom): 225.967,
p value: .5351.

Deviance chi-square fit statistic (based on 240 degrees of freedom): 251.965,
p value: .1593.

DEFINE CA5YRDPR:
EXP(-4.8291+4.3848*AGECUIRI-.5241*SITCUIRI+4.4029*SIZCUIRI+
4.8313*MITCUIRI)/[1+
EXP(-4.8291+4.3848*AGECUIRI-.5241*SITCUIRI+4.4029*SIZCUIRI+
4.8313*MITCUIRI)] IF FIRSTAGE#UNDEFS

The CA5YRDPR attribute assigns an individual probability of experiencing death
due to metastatic breast cancer within five years of diagnosis to each of the
677 patients based on the above four conventional breast cancer prognostic
factors converted by SPSA to corresponding UIRI values, but without any
consideration of AJCC stage at diagnosis. These 677 individual probabilities
were then subjected to a ROC/AUC analysis.

The area under the complete ROC curve was estimated to be 0.7872.

Converting the four conventional breast cancer prognostic factors to
corresponding UIRI values produced an improvement in AUC value of 0.0164, from
0.7708 to 0.7872, compared to the factor-centered base case analysis. The
statistical fit with the logistic regression model was roughly comparable. It
also produced an index of error reduction = 0.0960. A Wilcoxon test generated a
normalized Z statistic = 4.34, with a two-tail p value < 0.00005.

Compared to the practice-centered base case, however, the AUC value decreased
by 0.0141, from 0.8013 to 0.7872, resulting in a negative index of error
reduction = -0.0960 and a corresponding normalized Z statistic = -2.03, with a
two-tail p value = 0.0429.

The last analysis to be performed with no missing observations was designed to assess the incremental improvement in predictive accuracy realizable from stratifying patients into low-risk, medium-risk, and high-risk subgroups— given that UIRI indexes had been substituted for their corresponding conventional breast cancer prognostic factors as independent variable inputs to logistic regression. Three separate logistic regressions were executed, one on each risk subgroup. This required executing SPSA three times to produce, where possible, a UIRI value for each of the conventional breast cancer prognostic factors, separately, for each risk subgroup. To distinguish among them, AGELUIRI designated the UIRI for AGE in the low-risk subgroup, AGEMUIRI designated the UIRI for AGE in the medium-risk subgroup, and AGEHUIRI designated the UIRI for AGE in the high-risk subgroup. L, M, and H designators were also used to distinguish UIRI values among subgroups for the other four conventional breast cancer prognostic factors.

All three regression analyses generated highly significant likelihood ratio chi-square statistics. The three separate regression outputs are not shown below, but the expression used to merge the three sets of results into the definition of the CS5YRDPR attribute is displayed.

Notice that ULCLUIRI (the conventional breast cancer prognostic ulceration factor converted to a corresponding UIRI index for the low-risk subgroup), AGEMUIRI (the conventional age factor converted to a corresponding UIRI index for the medium-risk subgroup), ULCMUIRI (the conventional ulceration factor converted to a corresponding UIRI index for the medium-risk subgroup), and ULCHUIRI (the conventional breast cancer prognostic ulceration factor converted to a corresponding UIRI index for the high-risk subgroup) have been removed from the analysis. This is because the SPSA algorithm rejected all four of these UIRI indexes as either possessing too small a sample size or pointing in no direction or pointing in the wrong direction.

```
DEFINE CS5YRDPR:
EXP(-7.0705+12.5809*AGELUIRI+16.3428*SITLUIRI+10.7715*SIZLUIRI+
10.3240*MITLUIRI)/[1+
EXP(-7.0705+12.5809*AGELUIRI+16.3428*SITLUIRI+10.7715*SIZLUIRI+
10.3240*MITLUIRI)] IF
CONVAGE#UNDEFN AND CONVSITE#UNDEFN AND CONVSIZE#UNDEFN AND CONVMITC#UNDEFN
AND CONVULC#UNDEFN AND FIRSTAGE#UNDEFS AND RISKLEVL=LOWRISK ELSE
EXP(-4.5418+3.1175*SITMUIRI+3.8472*SIZMUIRI+5.0412*MITMUIRI)/[1+
EXP(-4.5418+3.1175*SITMUIRI+3.8472*SIZMUIRI+5.0412*MITMUIRI)] IF
CONVAGE#UNDEFN AND CONVSITE#UNDEFN AND CONVSIZE#UNDEFN AND CONVMITC#UNDEFN
AND CONVULC#UNDEFN AND FIRSTAGE#UNDEFS AND RISKLEVL=MEDRISK ELSE
EXP(-15.3829+6.9204*AGEHUIRI+5.2818*SITHUIRI+5.0670*SIZHUIRI+
4.8343*MITHUIRI)/[1+
EXP(-15.3829+6.9204*AGEHUIRI+5.2818*SITHUIRI+5.0670*SIZHUIRI+
4.8343*MITHUIRI)] IF
CONVAGE#UNDEFN AND CONVSITE#UNDEFN AND CONVSIZE#UNDEFN AND CONVMITC#UNDEFN
AND CONVULC#UNDEFN AND FIRSTAGE#UNDEFS AND RISKLEVL=HIGHRISK
```

The CS5YRDPR attribute assigns an individual probability of experiencing death due to metastatic breast cancer within five years of diagnosis to each of the 677 patients based on the above five conventional breast cancer prognostic factors converted, where possible, by SPSA to corresponding UIRI values— separately for each risk subgroup—but without using AJCC stage as an independent variable of logistic regression. These 677 individual probabilities were then subjected to a ROC/AUC analysis.

The area under the complete ROC curve was estimated to be 0.8754.

Just as in the melanoma analysis, stratifying patients into low-risk, medium-risk, and high-risk subgroups increased the AUC, this time by 0.0882, from 0.7872 to 0.8754, compared to simply converting conventional prognostic factors into corresponding UIRI values. It also produced an index of error reduction = 0.3944. A Wilcoxon test generated a normalized Z statistic = 10.36, with a two-tail p value < 0.00005. Compared to the practice-centered base case, the AUC increased equally dramatically by 0.0741, from 0.8013 to 0.8754, producing an index of error reduction = 0.3767. A Wilcoxon test generated a normalized Z statistic = 9.03, with a two-tail p value < 0.00005.

These results demonstrate that the combined impact of stratifying patients by risk subgroup and then substituting corresponding UIRI values for the admissible conventional breast cancer prognostic factors (separately by risk subgroup) again produced significantly more accurate individual probabilistic predictions (in terms of both AUC values and probabilistic prediction errors) than basing predictions solely on initial AJCC staging classification. Because none of the 677 breast cancer patients possessed any missing observations, these results cannot be attributed in any way to the somewhat unusual manner in which SPSA handles missing data.

4.3 Analysis of Traditional Prognostic Factors with Missing Observations

Once again we adopted as a conventional factor-centered base case the five routinely recorded breast cancer prognostic factors described in section 4.2. These included CONVAGE, CONVSITE, CONVSIZE, CONVMITC, AND CONVULC. There were no missing observations on either CONVAGE or CONVMITC. CONVSITE, CONVSIZE, and CONVULC all contained missing observations for at least some of the 1,225 patients.

Patients were not stratified according to their risk of experiencing disease-specific death within five years for this revised factor-centered base case analysis. What was different here was that no patients with missing observations were excluded from the analysis. Instead, they were treated in a commonly practiced factor-centered manner. Each missing observation was replaced by the mean of the nonmissing observations for that prognostic factor in the sample of 1,225 patients.

The results of a standard logistic regression on these five prognostic factors with missing observations replaced by mean values are shown below.

```
DEFINE CONVSITM: CONVSITE IF CONVSITE#UNDEFN ELSE MEAN(CONVSITE)
DEFINE CONVSIZM: CONVSIZE IF CONVSIZE#UNDEFN ELSE MEAN(CONVSIZE)
DEFINE CONVULCM: CONVULC IF CONVULC#UNDEFN ELSE MEAN(CONVULC)
```

RESULTS OF LOGISTIC REGRESSION ANALYSIS (LINEAR MODEL)

The dependent variable is a binary-coded numeric variable whose values are either 0 or 1. It is embodied in the first expression (parameter) of the LOGREG command, which is just the attribute DSSDUMMY.

The independent variable CONVAGE is just the attribute CONVAGE.
The independent variable CONVSITM is just the attribute CONVSITM.
The independent variable CONVSIZM is just the attribute CONVSIZM.
The independent variable CONVMITC is just the attribute CONVMITC.
The independent variable CONVULCM is just the attribute CONVULCM.

Likelihood ratio chi-square statistic: 234.963, two-tail p value: .0000 (based on 5 degrees of freedom and 1225 complete observations).

INDEPENDENT VARIABLE	REGRESSION COEFFICIENT	STANDARD DEVIATION	CHI-SQUARE (DF = 1)	2-TAIL P VALUE	ODDS RATIO MULTIPLIER
intercept	-3.3828	.3770	80.5233	.0000	.0340
CONVAGE	.0674	.0519	1.6850	.1943	1.0697
CONVSITM	.5982	.1802	11.0179	.0009	1.8189
CONVSIZM	.4657	.0824	31.9697	.0000	1.5931
CONVMITC	1.5176	.1510	101.0562	.0000	4.5613
CONVULCM	2.1341	.4695	20.6582	.0000	8.4494

GOODNESS OF STATISTICAL FIT OF LOGISTIC REGRESSION MODEL

Pearson chi-square fit statistic (based on 159 degrees of freedom): 220.946, p value: .0008.

Deviance chi-square fit statistic (based on 159 degrees of freedom): 241.283, p value: .0000.

[Technical note: Substituting mean values for missing observations required replacing CONVULC with CONVULCM in the analysis. This eliminated CONVULC's statistically unstable regression coefficient, but it reduced substantially the goodness of statistical fit of the logistic regression model.]

DEFINE N5YRDPR:
EXP(-3.3828+.0674*CONVAGE+.5982*CONVSITM+.4657*CONVSIZM+1.5176*CONVMITC+
2.1341*CONVULCM)/[1+
EXP(-3.3828+.0674*CONVAGE+.5982*CONVSITM+.4657*CONVSIZM+1.5176*CONVMITC+
2.1341*CONVULCM)]

The N5YRDPR attribute assigns an individual probability of experiencing death due to metastatic breast cancer within five years of diagnosis to each of the 1,225 patients based on the above five conventional breast cancer prognostic factors when each missing observation is replaced by the mean of the nonmissing observations for that prognostic factor. These 1,225 individual probabilities were then subjected to a ROC/AUC analysis.

The area under the complete ROC curve was estimated to be 0.7433.

Comparison of these results with those displayed in section 4.2 shows a reduction in AUC of 0.0275 from 0.7708 to 0.7433 and a substantially reduced goodness of statistical fit of the logistic regression model from treating missing observations in a typical factor-centered manner. There was, however, an increase in effective sample size from 677 to 1,225. That served to preserve chi-square and associated p values at quite respectable levels. The reduced AUC value of 0.7433 will become our revised factor-centered base case level for all subsequent comparisons that encompass missing observations.

The next revised analysis replicated the previous practice-centered base case logistic regression. The same dummy variables were used to represent the AJCC staging classification scheme. This time, however, the forty-eight patients with missing observations of initial AJCC stage were assigned five-year disease-specific death probabilities according to the incidence of that focal event among all patients with such missing observations in their risk subgroup.

RESULTS OF LOGISTIC REGRESSION ANALYSIS (LINEAR MODEL)

The dependent variable is a binary-coded numeric variable whose values are either 0 or 1. It is embodied in the first expression (parameter) of the LOGREG command, which is just the attribute DSSDUMMY.

The independent variable EXPRESSION2 is 1 IF FIRSTAGE="0" ELSE 0.
The independent variable EXPRESSION3 is 1 IF FIRSTAGE="1a" OR "1b" ELSE 0.
The independent variable EXPRESSION4 is 1 IF FIRSTAGE="2a" ELSE 0.
The independent variable EXPRESSION5 is 1 IF FIRSTAGE="2b" ELSE 0.
The independent variable EXPRESSION6 is 1 IF FIRSTAGE="3a" ELSE 0.
The independent variable EXPRESSION7 is 1 IF FIRSTAGE="3b" ELSE 0.
The independent variable EXPRESSION8 is 1 IF FIRSTAGE="4" ELSE 0.

Likelihood ratio chi-square statistic: 388.268, two-tail p value: .0000 (based on 7 degrees of freedom and 1225 complete observations).

INDEPENDENT VARIABLE	REGRESSION COEFFICIENT	STANDARD DEVIATION	CHI-SQUARE (DF = 1)	2-TAIL P VALUE	ODDS RATIO MULTIPLIER
intercept	-.4568	.2932	2.4269	.1193	.6333
EXPRESSION2	-11.8527	271.8956	.0019	.9652	.0000
EXPRESSION3	-2.3335	.4022	33.6592	.0000	.0970
EXPRESSION4	-1.3821	.3413	16.4020	.0001	.2510
EXPRESSION5	-.1411	.4763	.0877	.7671	.8684
EXPRESSION6	.4802	.3088	2.4186	.1199	1.6164
EXPRESSION7	.9110	.3561	6.5434	.0105	2.4868
EXPRESSION8	2.8200	.4719	35.7035	.0000	16.7763

[Technical notes: Seven zero-one dummy variables served as the independent variables. The forty-eight patients whose initial AJCC stage was undetermined were assigned zero values on all seven dummy variables. All patients initially diagnosed in stage 3c died within five years of MBC. They were, likewise, assigned zero values on all seven dummy variables. Eleven of thirty low-risk patients, six of seventeen medium-risk patients, and the one high-risk patient whose AJCC stage could not be determined died of MBC within five years.]

DEFINE F5YRDPR:
EXP(-.4568-11.8527)/[1+EXP(-.4568-11.8527)] IF FIRSTAGE="0" ELSE
EXP(-.4568-2.3335)/[1+EXP(-.4568-2.3335)] IF FIRSTAGE="1a" OR "1b" ELSE
EXP(-.4568-1.3821)/[1+EXP(-.4568-1.3821)] IF FIRSTAGE="2a" ELSE
EXP(-.4568-.1411)/[1+EXP(-.4568-.1411)] IF FIRSTAGE="2b" ELSE
EXP(-.4568+.4802)/[1+EXP(-.4568+.4802)] IF FIRSTAGE="3a" ELSE
EXP(-.4568+.9110)/[1+EXP(-.4568+.9110)] IF FIRSTAGE="3b" ELSE
EXP(-.4568+2.8200)/[1+EXP(-.4568+2.8200)] IF FIRSTAGE="4" ELSE
1.0000 IF FIRSTAGE="3c" ELSE
11/30 IF RISKLEVL=LOWRISK ELSE
6/17 IF RISKLEVL=MEDRISK ELSE
1/1 IF RISKLEVL=HIGHRISK

The F5YRDPR attribute assigns an individual probability of experiencing death due to metastatic breast cancer within five years of diagnosis to each of the 1,225 patients based solely on AJCC stage at diagnosis as a classificatory (dummy-variable) input to logistic regression. When initial AJCC stage could not be determined, patients were assigned five-year disease-specific death probabilities according to the incidence of that focal event among all patients with such missing observations in their risk subgroup. These 1,225 individual probabilities were then subjected to a ROC/AUC analysis.

The area under the complete ROC curve was estimated to be 0.8021.

Substituting the initial AJCC staging classification for the five conventional breast cancer factors increased the AUC by 0.0588, from 0.7433 to 0.8021. It also produced an index of error reduction = 0.3143 compared to the revised factor-centered base case analysis. A Wilcoxon test was performed on the 1,225 matched pairs of probabilistic prediction errors, showing a normalized Z statistic = 7.57, with a two-tail p value < 0.00005.

Each prognostic factor's optimal scale partitioning and numeric rescaling is embodied in its univariate impact-reflecting index (UIRI) produced by the Scale Partitioning and Spacing Algorithm (SPSA). The five UIRI variables were substituted for their corresponding five conventional breast cancer prognostic factors, and the following logistic regression analysis was performed.

RESULTS OF LOGISTIC REGRESSION ANALYSIS (LINEAR MODEL)

The dependent variable is a binary-coded numeric variable whose values are either 0 or 1. It is embodied in the first expression (parameter) of the LOGREG command, which is just the attribute DSSDUMMY.

The independent variable AGEAUIRI is just the attribute AGEAUIRI.
The independent variable SITAUIRI is just the attribute SITAUIRI.
The independent variable SIZAUIRI is just the attribute SIZAUIRI.
The independent variable MITAUIRI is just the attribute MITAUIRI.
The independent variable ULCAUIRI is just the attribute ULCAUIRI.

Likelihood ratio chi-square statistic: 333.494, two-tail p value: .0000 (based on 5 degrees of freedom and 1225 complete observations).

INDEPENDENT VARIABLE	REGRESSION COEFFICIENT	STANDARD DEVIATION	CHI-SQUARE (DF = 1)	2-TAIL P VALUE	ODDS RATIO MULTIPLIER
intercept	−7.5480	.7056	114.4189	.0000	.0005
AGEAUIRI	4.7897	1.3989	11.7235	.0006	120.2701
SITAUIRI	2.1723	.7465	8.4689	.0036	8.7787
SIZAUIRI	4.0463	.4625	76.5488	.0000	57.1871
MITAUIRI	4.4188	.4187	111.3836	.0000	83.0002
ULCAUIRI	3.3126	.9308	12.6668	.0004	27.4577

GOODNESS OF STATISTICAL FIT OF LOGISTIC REGRESSION MODEL

Pearson chi-square fit statistic (based on 255 degrees of freedom): 290.489, p value: .0626.

Deviance chi-square fit statistic (based on 255 degrees of freedom): 286.347, p value: .0863.

DEFINE A5YRDPR:
EXP(−7.5480+4.7897*AGEAUIRI+2.1723*SITAUIRI+4.0463 *SIZAUIRI+4.4188*MITAUIRI+ 3.3126*ULCAUIRI)/[1+
EXP(−7.5480+4.7897*AGEAUIRI+2.1723*SITAUIRI+4.0463 *SIZAUIRI+4.4188*MITAUIRI+ 3.3126*ULCAUIRI)]

The A5YRDPR attribute assigns an individual probability of experiencing death due to metastatic breast cancer within five years of diagnosis to each of the 1,225 patients based on the above five conventional breast cancer prognostic factors converted by SPSA to corresponding UIRI values, but without using AJCC stage at diagnosis as an independent variable of logistic regression. These 1,225 individual probabilities were then subjected to a ROC/AUC analysis.

The area under the complete ROC curve was estimated to be 0.7963.

Converting the five conventional breast cancer prognostic factors to corresponding UIRI indexes improved the AUC value by 0.0530, from 0.7433 to 0.7963, compared to the revised factor-centered base case analysis. It also produced an index of error reduction = 0.2392. A Wilcoxon test generated a normalized Z statistic = 8.90, with a two-tail p value < 0.00005.

Compared to the practice-centered base case, however, the AUC value declined by 0.0058, from 0.8021 to 0.7963. Despite the small decline, this still produced a positive index of error reduction = 0.0743. A Wilcoxon test also generated a positive normalized Z statistic = 1.87, with a two-tail p value = 0.0620.

When a prognostic factor is dichotomous, simply substituting a corresponding UIRI index as an independent variable of logistic regression produces no predictive improvement. Anatomical location of primary tumor and ulceration are conventionally treated as possessing only two possible data values each.

Regrettably, the breast cancer data set coded mitotic rate (MITCOUNT) only trichotomously. This may explain, in part, why the A5YRDPR individual patient probabilities provided less improvement than the corresponding A5YRDPR probabilities in the melanoma analysis.

Excluding the way SPSA handles missing observations, the predictive improvement produced by defining the A5YRDPR attribute is, therefore, mostly attributable to patient age and primary tumor size. Figures 12 and 13 show substitute UIRI scattergrams for these two conventional prognostic factors.

Comparing Figure 12 with Figure 2 suggests that the impact of age at diagnosis on disease-specific death is similar in both melanoma and breast cancer, except at rather young ages. The shapes of the two UIRI scattergrams are strikingly similar, except when a melanoma patient is diagnosed before reaching the age of thirty. The "low tail" of the melanoma scattergram is not reproduced in the breast cancer scattergram—perhaps because breast cancer patients in the Turku training sample were rarely diagnosed at an age below forty.

Figure 3 suggests that the impact of primary tumor thickness on MM death in melanoma increases steadily, but at a steadily decreasing rate. Figure 13 suggests that the impact of primary tumor size on MBC death in breast cancer also increases steadily, but at a more or less constant rate.

The analysis that produced A5YRDPR did not provide a very good statistical fit with the logistic regression model. Both the Pearson chi-square and the deviance chi-square statistics suggested that the model might reasonably be rejected. Fortunately, the logistic regression model did fit the data quite well in the next analysis when patients were stratified by risk group.

The last analysis of conventional prognostic factors was designed to assess the incremental improvement in predictive accuracy realizable from stratifying patients into low-risk, medium-risk, and high-risk subgroups—given that the five UIRI indexes had been substituted for their corresponding five conventional breast cancer prognostic factors as independent variables of logistic regression. Three separate logistic regressions were executed, one on each risk subgroup. This required executing SPSA three times to produce a UIRI value for each of the five conventional breast cancer prognostic factors, separately, for each risk subgroup.

Figure 12

Scattergram of UIRI for Age at Initial Diagnosis

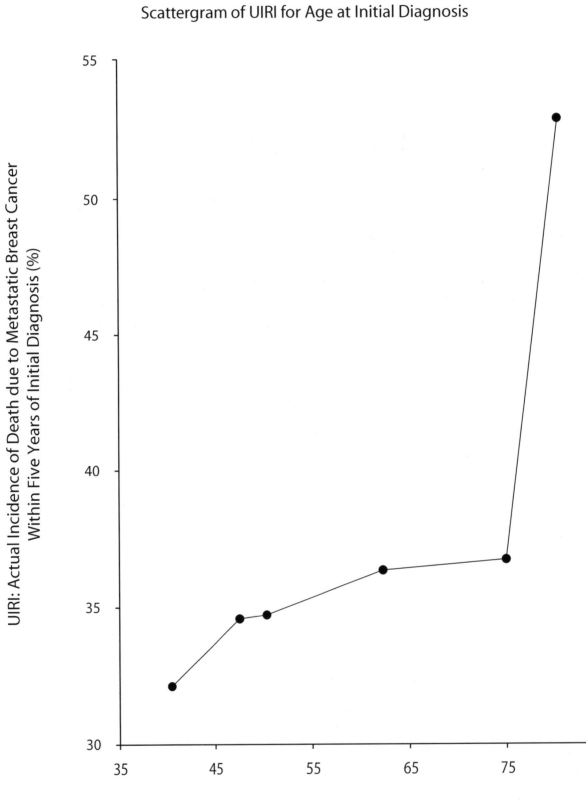

Mean Age at Initial Diagnosis (years)

Figure 13

Scattergram of UIRI for Size of Primary Tumor

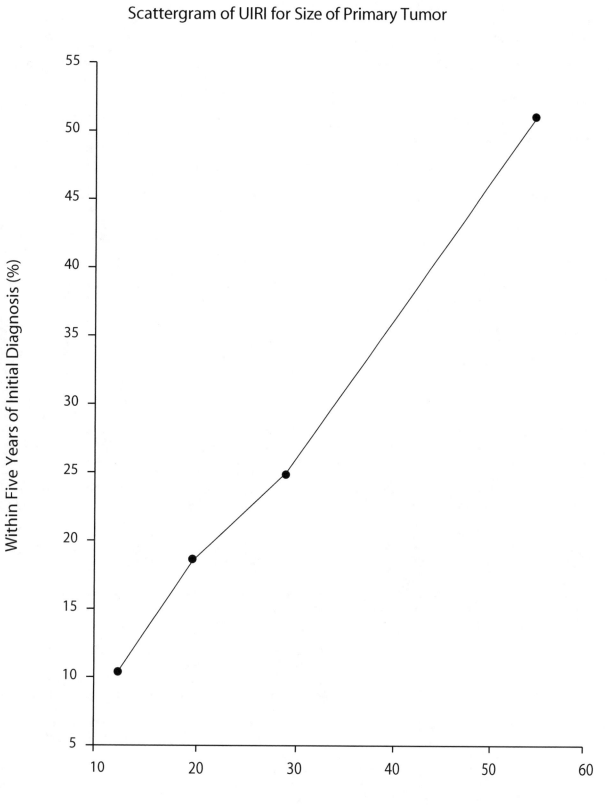

UIRI: Actual Incidence of Death due to Metastatic Breast Cancer Within Five Years of Initial Diagnosis (%)

Mean Size of Primary Tumor (mm)

All three regression analyses generated highly significant likelihood ratio chi-square statistics. The three separate regression outputs are not shown below, nor is the expression used to merge the three sets of results into the combined attribute, S5YRDPR. The same outputs and procedures were illustrated in the previous analysis of 677 breast cancer patients with no missing observations. The 1,225 individual probabilities calculated for S5YRDPR (which accounts for missing observations) were then subjected to a ROC/AUC analysis.

The area under the complete ROC curve was estimated to be 0.8792.

S5YRDPR did provide a quite reasonable statistical fit with the logistic regression model, as shown below.

GOODNESS OF STATISTICAL FIT OF LOGISTIC REGRESSION MODEL

Pearson chi-square fit statistic (based on 285 degrees of freedom): 277.463, p value: .6143.

Deviance chi-square fit statistic (based on 285 degrees of freedom): 269.719, p value: .7336.

Stratifying patients into low-risk, medium-risk, and high-risk subgroups and converting conventional prognostic factors to corresponding UIRI values improved predictive accuracy relative to all three revised analyses. This combined procedure increased the AUC by 0.0771, from 0.8021 to 0.8792, compared to the practice-centered base case, which generated the most accurate of the three revised predictions. It also produced an index of error reduction = 0.3649. A Wilcoxon test generated a normalized Z statistic = 11.87, with a two-tail p value < 0.00005.

S5YRDPR embodies our proposed PCM approach when applied just to the five conventional breast cancer prognostic factors. We must demonstrate once more that combining the predictive information contained in the N5YRDPR attribute with the (partially overlapping) information contained in the F5YRDPR attribute in the PCM manner produces more accurate individually tailored five-year disease-specific death predictions than if the same information were combined via standard logistic regression. This is accomplished in the next paragraph.

In section 4.1, the five conventional breast cancer factors and the equivalent of F5YRDPR (both without missing observations) served as inputs to a standard logistic regression analysis. This time, N5YRDPR was substituted for the five conventional factors. When combined with F5YRDPR as a second independent variable, the resulting logistic regression accounted for all missing data. Its output was converted, as usual, to individual MBC death probabilities and labeled NF5YRDPR.

1. A ROC analysis of NF5YRDPR produced an AUC of 0.8468. This constituted an AUC increase of 0.1035 compared to N5YRDPR, with a corresponding index of error reduction = 0.4106. It produced a normalized Z statistic = 12.88, significant at two-tail p < 0.00005 via a Wilcoxon test.
2. It also constituted an AUC increase of 0.0447 compared to F5YRDPR, with a corresponding index of error reduction = 0.2180. It produced a normalized Z statistic = 8.43, significant at two-tail p < 0.00005 via a Wilcoxon test.
3. Most important, our PCM approach (S5YRDPR) produced an AUC of 0.8792. This constituted an AUC increase of 0.0324 compared to NF5YRDPR, with a corresponding index of error reduction = 0.2947. It produced a normalized Z statistic = 9.14, significant at two-tail p < 0.00005 via a Wilcoxon test.

All of these results show that our PCM approach produced significantly more accurate individual probabilistic predictions (in terms of both AUC values and probabilistic prediction errors) than any of the other prognostic methodologies, including the commonly practiced procedure of basing predictions solely on initial AJCC staging classification. Also, the manner in which SPSA handles missing observations again seemed to enhance rather than to dilute the accuracy improvement realized in the absence of missing observations.

4.4 Adding Nontraditional Prognostic Factors to the Analysis

Two groups of nontraditional prognostic factors were then added to the five conventional factors in predicting MBC death within five years for the 1,225 breast cancer patients.

Nontraditional here simply means not included among the five conventional prognostic factors defined in the factor-centered base case analysis. Observations on the T, N, and M scales, for example, although frequently made, were not classified as conventional. They were classified as nontraditional to facilitate comparability of results with the melanoma analysis.

The first nontraditional group included the following twelve (histological) factors, all of which were ascertainable at the time of initial diagnosis:

1. primary tumor's histological subtype (lobular versus ductal)—risk higher when ductal;
2. grade of primary tumor (1 = low grade versus 2 = medium grade versus 3 = high grade, where assignment of grade depends, in part, on mitotic count)—risk increases with higher grade;
3. degree of necrosis (1 = none versus 2 = spotty versus 3 = moderate versus 4 = severe)—risk increases with higher degree of necrosis;
4. extent of tubule formation (1 = extensive versus 2 = moderate versus 3 = slight or none)—risk decreases with higher extent of tubule formation;
5. degree of nuclear pleomorphism (1 = slight versus 2 = moderate versus 3 = severe)—risk increases with greater degree of pleomorphism;
6. inflammatory cancer (0 = no versus 1 = yes)—risk higher when inflammatory;
7. estrogen receptor (ER, measured in fmol./mg.)—risk decreases with higher measured ER level;
8. progesterone receptor (PR, measured in fmol./mg.)—risk decreases with higher measured PR level;
9. bilaterality (0 = no versus 1 = yes)—risk decreases when bilateral;
10. T (tumor characteristic) scale (0 = T0 versus 1 = T1 versus 2 = T2 versus 3 = T3 versus 4 = T4)—risk increases with higher T scale value;
11. N (nodal involvement) scale (0 = N0 for none versus 1 = N1 versus 2 = N2 versus 3 = N3)—risk increases with higher N scale value; and
12. M (metastasis) scale (0 = M0 for nonmetastatic versus 1 = M1 for metastatic)—risk increases when diagnosed metastatic (1 = M1).

The second nontraditional group included two therapeutic factors, typically determined shortly after the time of initial diagnosis. These two factors were:

1. radiation therapy (0 = no versus 1 = yes)—risk decreases when patient receives radiation therapy; and
2. adjuvant therapy (see appendix D for a list of therapies offered).

Based on the prediction improvements already achieved for the five conventional prognostic factors, the twelve factors in the first nontraditional group were first converted by SPSA to corresponding UIRI values exactly as previously described, and the composite collection of seventeen converted UIRI factors was then subjected to three separate logistic regression analyses, one for each of the three risk subgroups of breast cancer patients. The results of the three separate logistic regressions were merged into a composite attribute called G15YRDPR, also in the same manner as previously described. The 1,225 individual probabilities calculated for G15YRDPR (which accounts for missing observations of both the five conventional and the twelve nontraditional factors in the first group) were then subjected to a ROC/AUC analysis.

The area under the complete ROC curve was estimated to be 0.8986.

Adding the new histological information encapsulated within the twelve factors in the first nontraditional group to the five conventional factors increased the AUC by 0.0194, from 0.8792 achieved by S5YRDPR to 0.8986 achieved by G15YRDPR, and increased to a very high level the goodness of statistical fit of the logistic regression model. It also produced an index of error reduction = 0.3159. A Wilcoxon test generated a normalized Z statistic = 10.22, with a two-tail p value < 0.00005.

The two therapeutic factors in the second nontraditional group were then converted by SPSA to corresponding UIRI values exactly as previously described, and the composite collection of nineteen converted UIRI factors was subjected to three separate logistic regression analyses, one for each of the three risk subgroups of breast cancer patients. The results of the three separate logistic regressions were merged into a composite attribute called G25YRDPR, also in the same manner as previously described. The 1,225 individual probabilities calculated for G25YRDPR (which accounts for missing observations of the five conventional factors, the twelve histological factors in the first nontraditional group, and the two therapeutic factors in the second nontraditional group) were then subjected to a ROC/AUC analysis.

The area under the complete ROC curve was estimated to be 0.9003.

Adding the new therapeutic information encapsulated within the two factors in the second nontraditional group to the five conventional breast cancer factors and the twelve histological factors in the first nontraditional group increased the AUC by 0.0017, from 0.8986 achieved by G15YRDPR to 0.9003 achieved by G25YRDPR, while still preserving at the same very high level the goodness of statistical fit of the logistic regression model. It also produced an index of error reduction = 0.1902. A Wilcoxon test generated a normalized Z statistic = 3.83, with a two-tail p value = 0.0001.

4.5 How Selection Bias Can Severely Distort the Apparent Efficacy of Therapy

Our patient-centered analysis of the consequences of receiving adjuvant therapy provided some striking insights.

The table on the next page shows that 807 of the breast cancer patients in the Turku sample received no adjuvant therapy, while thirty-one patients received Tamoxifen.

VALUE OF ATTRIBUTE ADJUVNTX	VALUE OF ATTRIBUTE DSS5YR		
	DSS>5YRS	MBC DEATH=<5YRS	TOTAL
NO ADJUVANT THERAPY	494	313	807
TAMOXIFEN	15	16	31
TOTAL	509	329	838

Without using initial AJCC stage to stratify patients into risk subgroups and without controlling for surgery and radiation therapy received, the table suggests that patients who received Tamoxifen were more likely to experience MBC death within five years of diagnosis (16 of 31 = 51.61 percent) than patients who received no adjuvant therapy (313 of 807 = 38.79 percent).

This seems counterintuitive. Is it possible that receiving Tamoxifen actually compromised the survival of those thirty-one Turku patients?

The time elapsed until MBC death was then compared between these two groups via a Kaplan-Meier analysis. Yes, patients who received Tamoxifen also tended to survive for a shorter period, and the difference in survival times was statistically significant (Log-rank test two-tail p value = 0.0211, Figure 14).

A possible explanation of these anomalous results is substantial selection bias.

When it first became available, Tamoxifen was selectively administered to the "sicker" patients in the Turku training sample (i.e., to patients at later stages of disease progression when diagnosed). None of the thirty-one patients who received Tamoxifen were in the low-risk subgroup. All thirty-one were in the medium-risk and high-risk subgroups.

By matching patients according both to AJCC stage at diagnosis and to type of surgery and according to whether or not they received radiation therapy, this selection bias was effectively removed from the analysis. The impact of receiving versus not receiving Tamoxifen was uniformly compared between separate members of thirty-one pairs of patients matched as just described. Then, the significant benefit of Tamoxifen (longer, rather than shorter survival times until MBC death) clearly emerged. It overcame the substantial selection bias that initially masked it (Wilcoxon matched-pairs, signed-ranks test two-tail p value = 0.0046; binomial sign test two-tail p value = 0.0241).

Strict eligibility criteria and other control mechanisms eliminate this problem from carefully designed clinical trials. However, in retrospective analyses such as this, matching and other statistical devices are essential to avoid drawing dramatically misleading conclusions.

Most of the Turku patients (75.02 percent) received radiation therapy. No selection bias occurred in assessing its efficacy. Radiation appeared to prolong survival time, as anticipated.

Figure 14

Kaplan-Meier Survival Analysis

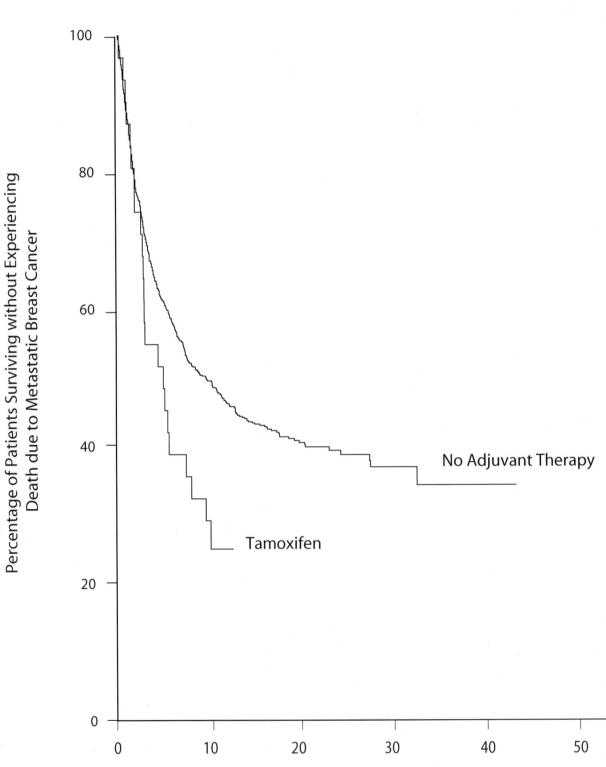

4.6   Summary of Breast Cancer Results

Adding fourteen nontraditional prognostic factors to five conventional factors, with all nineteen factors analyzed according to the patient-centered methodology, produced the following improvements in predictive accuracy.

1. Compared to the conventional factor-centered base case, AUC increased by 15.70 percentage points, from 74.33 percent to 90.03 percent. This was a more dramatic improvement than in the case of melanoma. The maximum achievable percentage of correct predictions increased by 13.55 points, from 69.39 percent to 82.94 percent. This, too, was a more dramatic improvement than in the case of melanoma.
2. Compared to the practice-centered base case, AUC increased by 9.82 percentage points, from 80.21 percent to 90.03 percent. This was a more dramatic improvement than in the case of melanoma. The maximum achievable percentage of correct predictions increased by 10.61 points, from 72.33 percent to 82.94 percent. This, too, was a more dramatic improvement than in the case of melanoma.
3. All of these increases compare even more favorably than in the case of the comparable melanoma results with the meager, two-percentage-point improvement reported by Dr. Ware in 2006, where statistically significant nontraditional prognostic factors were added to conventional factors—but without the benefit of our proposed patient-centered methodology.
4. As measured by the index of error reduction and the Wilcoxon matched-pairs, signed-ranks tests, these improvements were highly significant, all showing two-tail p values < 0.00005.

PCM analysis of breast cancer patients supported another disarmingly simple and accurate prediction.

Suppose that any patient who appeared at least as likely as not to die of metastatic breast cancer within five years of diagnosis (i.e., any patient whose individually tailored composite G25YRDPR probability was at least 50 percent) were predicted to experience that calamity, while all other patients were predicted to survive for more than five years. For what percentage of the 1,225 patients in our training sample would these have been correct predictions? The relative frequency table on the next page shows this to be 0.5616 + 0.2645 = 82.61 percent. This is very nearly as high as the maximum possible hit rate of 82.94 percent.

TABLE OF JOINT ABSOLUTE FREQUENCIES (COUNTS)

VALUE OF FIRST EXPRESSION	VALUE OF ATTRIBUTE DSS5YR		
	DSS>5YRS	MBC DEATH=<5YRS	TOTAL
PREDICT DSS>5YRS	688	122	810
PREDICT MBC DEATH=<5YRS	91	324	415
TOTAL	779	446	1225

TABLE OF JOINT RELATIVE FREQUENCIES (PROPORTIONS)

VALUE OF FIRST EXPRESSION	VALUE OF ATTRIBUTE DSS5YR		
	DSS>5YRS	MBC DEATH=<5YRS	TOTAL
PREDICT DSS>5YRS	.5616	.0996	.6612
PREDICT MBC DEATH=<5YRS	.0743	.2645	.3388
TOTAL	.6359	.3641	1.0000

We must acknowledge that basing predictions on the 50 percent individually tailored probability does not always work this well. That it worked so well for our 1,225 breast cancer patients depended, in large part, on their particular distribution of MBC death versus five-year DSS. The cut point that maximized the rate of correct predictions just happened to fall very near 50 percent.

Shown below are summary statistics for the individual patient probabilities of experiencing death due to metastatic breast cancer within five years of diagnosis produced by the six logistic regression analyses (N5YRDPR, A5YRDPR, F5YRDPR, S5YRDPR, G15YRDPR, and G25YRDPR).

Notice once again that the mean probabilities are all identical and equal to the incidence of death due to MBC among these 1,225 patients. Notice also the differences in the minimum to maximum ranges and the standard deviations of these individual probabilities. Not only does G25YRDPR produce the most accurate probabilistic predictions (as just shown in terms of AUC, maximum achievable percentage of correct predictions, and probabilistic prediction error), it also tends to "spread out" its probabilistic predictions more widely than all of the other five probabilistic logistic regression outputs. Finer discrimination is achieved in combination with greater accuracy, not at the expense of greater accuracy.

SUMMARY STATISTICS	ATTRIBUTE DSSDUMMY	
n DEFINED	1225	
MINIMUM	0	DSSDUMMY = 0 means survival for more than five years.
MEDIAN	0	
MAXIMUM	1	DSSDUMMY = 1 means MBC death within five years.
MEAN	.3641	
STD. DEV.	.4812	

SUMMARY STATISTICS	ATTRIBUTE N5YRDPR	ATTRIBUTE A5YRDPR	ATTRIBUTE F5YRDPR	ATTRIBUTE S5YRDPR	ATTRIBUTE G15YRDPR	ATTRIBUTE G25YRDPR
n DEFINED	1225	1225	1225	1225	1225	1225
MINIMUM	.0621	.0372	.0000	.0099	.0044	.0055
MEDIAN	.4089	.3001	.5059	.2733	.2207	.2285
MAXIMUM	.9634	.9809	1.0000	.9896	.9982	.9990
MEAN	.3641	.3641	.3641	.3641	.3641	.3641
STD. DEV.	.2031	.2416	.2574	.3140	.3338	.3357

G25YRDPR was again the most accurate predictor in all of the senses previously discussed. Investigation of its scale characteristics throughout its complete logical range from zero to one will reveal other senses in which its probabilistic predictions were also remarkably reliable.

As in the case of melanoma, the 1,225 G25YRDPR individually tailored probabilities were first ranked and divided into quartiles. The mean of the probabilities in each quartile was then compared with the actual incidence of MBC death within five years of diagnosis among the patients in that quartile.

By virtue of the same convergence process discussed in the context of the United States Weather Bureau these two numbers should be about the same in each quartile. The maximum absolute difference was 1.49 percentage points. The mean absolute difference was 0.98 percentage points. Furthermore, there was no discernible pattern or trend in the succession of quartiles.

There were 1,082 distinctly different MBC death probability values of G25YRDPR for breast cancer patients. Consequently, we can investigate its scale characteristics more thoroughly—just as we did with melanoma.

The SPSA algorithm was executed to partition the scale of G25YRDPR into as many subscales as possible, as long as each subscale encompassed MBC death probabilities for at least twenty-five patients. Sixteen separate subscales were produced. They are shown below as SPSA's printed output. The corresponding actual incidence of MBC death within five years of diagnosis is shown as a fraction for each subscale.

```
0/78 IF G25YRDPR<.018 ELSE
1/70 IF G25YRDPR>=.018 AND G25YRDPR<.0307 ELSE
7/164 IF G25YRDPR>=.0307 AND G25YRDPR<.0648 ELSE
7/99 IF G25YRDPR>=.0648 AND G25YRDPR<.0981 ELSE
14/99 IF G25YRDPR>=.0981 AND G25YRDPR<.1522 ELSE
14/80 IF G25YRDPR>=.1522 AND G25YRDPR<.2104 ELSE
9/36 IF G25YRDPR>=.2104 AND G25YRDPR<.2402 ELSE
23/89 IF G25YRDPR>=.2402 AND G25YRDPR<.3555 ELSE
25/55 IF G25YRDPR>=.3555 AND G25YRDPR<.4249 ELSE
48/95 IF G25YRDPR>=.4249 AND G25YRDPR<.5788 ELSE
67/107 IF G25YRDPR>=.5788 AND G25YRDPR<.7433 ELSE
23/29 IF G25YRDPR>=.7433 AND G25YRDPR<.778 ELSE
28/34 IF G25YRDPR>=.778 AND G25YRDPR<.8346 ELSE
48/54 IF G25YRDPR>=.8346 AND G25YRDPR<.8993 ELSE
43/47 IF G25YRDPR>=.8993 AND G25YRDPR<.9545 ELSE
89/89 IF G25YRDPR>=.9545
```

The table below was then constructed. Prediction errors were calculated for each successive subscale as the mean of the G25YRDPR values falling within that subscale subtracted from the actual incidence of MBC death within five years among the at least twenty-five patients possessing those values of G25YRDPR.

SUBSCALE	LOWER AND UPPER SUBSCALE BOUNDS		SUBSCALE MEAN	ACTUAL INCIDENCE	PREDICTION ERROR
1	.0000 to	.0180	.0125	.0000	-.0125
2	.0180 to	.0307	.0241	.0143	-.0098
3	.0307 to	.0648	.0465	.0427	-.0038
4	.0648 to	.0981	.0794	.0707	-.0087
5	.0981 to	.1522	.1227	.1414	.0187
6	.1522 to	.2104	.1790	.1750	-.0040
7	.2104 to	.2402	.2258	.2500	.0242
8	.2402 to	.3555	.2867	.2584	-.0283
9	.3555 to	.4249	.3867	.4545	.0678
10	.4249 to	.5788	.5042	.5053	.0011
11	.5788 to	.7433	.6675	.6262	-.0413
12	.7433 to	.7780	.7557	.7931	.0374

13	.7780 to .8346	.8063	.8235	.0172
14	.8346 to .8993	.8668	.8889	.0221
15	.8993 to .9545	.9309	.9149	-.0160
16	.9545 to 1.0000	.9804	1.0000	.0196

Since the number of subscales expanded from four (quartiles) to sixteen, subscales contained fewer patient probabilities (between 29 and 164 each). Therefore, the convergence process was rendered less complete. The maximum absolute difference between the sixteen subscale means and their corresponding actual incidences was 6.78 percentage points. The mean absolute difference was 2.08 percentage points.

Taking algebraic signs into account, the mean prediction error should be very close to zero. It was 0.52 percentage points. Both a one-sample T test and a corresponding Wilcoxon test suggested that the population of prediction errors from which this sample of sixteen was drawn differed insignificantly from one with a mean and a median of zero.

When successive subscale means were plotted along the horizontal X-axis and the corresponding actual incidences were plotted along the vertical Y-axis of a graph, all sixteen points fell close to the straight line through the origin that makes a 45-degree angle with each axis. This line assumes that every actual incidence exactly equals its corresponding subscale mean. Prediction errors are vertical deviations from the line. The R squared value associated with this line, interpreted as a simple linear regression equation, was 0.9942 (equivalent to a 0.9971 linear correlation coefficient).

Detailed inspection of the sequence of prediction errors revealed no obvious patterns of any kind. There should be about as many positive errors as negative errors. There were eight positive and eight negative errors. There should be neither too many nor too few runs of sequential positive or negative signs. The intermediate number realized was about right, indicating randomness. The signed and absolute magnitudes of the prediction errors neither rose nor fell consistently. Relatively large and relatively small prediction errors clustered neither at the extremes of the probability scale nor in its interior.

Based on these observations, it seems appropriate to conclude that individually tailored G25YRDPR probabilities provide quite accurate predictions of whether or not a breast cancer patient will experience MBC death within five years of initial diagnosis. Figure 15 provides visual evidence of their predictive accuracy.

Figure 16 displays the four most salient ROC plots resulting from the breast cancer analysis:

1. the ROC plot based on the factor-centered base case analysis of the five conventional breast cancer prognostic factors, analyzed in the usual, factor-centered manner (N5YRDPR);
2. the ROC plot based on the practice-centered base case analysis—a dummy-variable logistic regression of initial AJCC stage alone (F5YRDPR);
3. the ROC plot based on the same five conventional prognostic factors, but now analyzed via our proposed patient-centered methodology, which uses AJCC stage at initial diagnosis as a stratifying variable for logistic regression and uniformly substitutes UIRI values for all prognostic factors (S5YRDPR); and
4. the ROC plot based on adding fourteen nontraditional factors to the same five conventional prognostic factors, again analyzed via the complete patient-centered methodology (G25YRDPR).

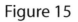

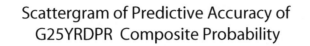

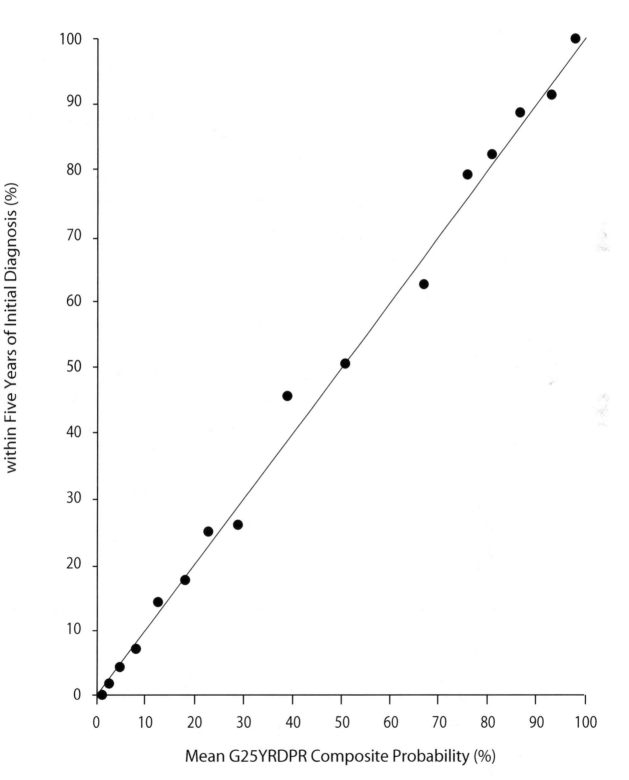

Figure 15

Scattergram of Predictive Accuracy of
G25YRDPR Composite Probability

Figure 16

ROC Analyses

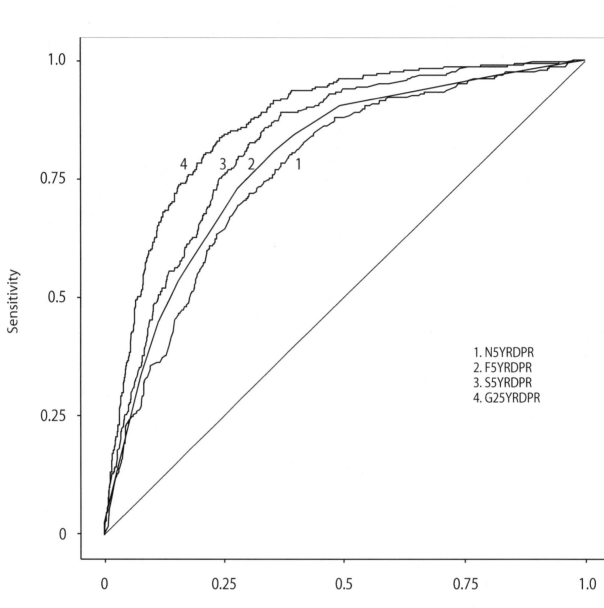

1. N5YRDPR
2. F5YRDPR
3. S5YRDPR
4. G25YRDPR

Section 2.8 described how to weight the relative predictive potency of the five conventional prognostic factors, the twelve nontraditional histological factors, and the two nontraditional therapeutic factors. These weights are tabled in appendix E.

The weight assigned to any factor in a risk subgroup (column of appendix E) indicates the predictive potency of that factor relative to the other factors in the same factor group. Hence, the weights add to 1.0 in each factor group and risk subgroup combination (nine combinations in all).

The explanatory notes in appendix E provide additional information on relative predictive potency weights across factor groups within separate risk subgroups. Such information would be useful in deciding exactly what additional prognostic factor information might prove most beneficial for a freshly diagnosed patient with less than complete readings on all nineteen factors (i.e., for almost all patients).

Appendix E suggests that the relative predictive potency of separate prognostic factors varies markedly across risk subgroups. The 1,225 breast cancer patients in the Turku training sample cannot be viewed as having been drawn from a single population, homogeneous in this sense. When such heterogeneity is detected, PCM exploits it by stratifying the training sample into separate risk subgroups and repeating the analysis, separately, for each risk subgroup.

There were three commonalities across risk subgroups. Mitotic count, tumor grade, and radiation therapy were assigned nonzero weights in all three risk subgroups. No other prognostic factors were.

5.0   CONCLUSIONS AND RECOMMENDATIONS

What has been presented so far should be regarded as proof of concept. The concept is making a transition from being factor-centered to becoming patient-centered in the prognosis of a progressive disease such as cancer.

Becoming patient-centered means at least the following things.

1. Drawing tailored prognostic conclusions separately applicable to individual patients becomes the ultimate methodological goal. Making generic statements about prognostic factors generalizable to some broadly defined patient population remains important, but its role in the patient-centered context is penultimate. Precisely this goal enhancement is the motivation for continuing to steps eight, nine, and ten, as outlined in section 1.1, rather than proceeding only through step seven.

2. Enhancing the goal in this manner has several implications. To begin with, it interchanges the means-ends relationship between using factor data to draw individually tailored conclusions about patients and using individual patient data to draw conclusions about separate prognostic factors. This interchange has a number of consequences.

3. One major consequence is to reinterpret what it means for a sample of empirical observations to be representative. It is no longer sufficient just to be population-based. It may even be inappropriate. In the patient-centered context, being population-based may serve the penultimate goal, but not necessarily the ultimate goal. To be representative now means to be specifically applicable to supporting accurate predictions relating to a targeted individual patient. This strongly suggests regularly reconceiving the fundamental concept of a patient population in stratified terms. Equally strongly, it suggests determining the appropriate principle of stratification, separately, on the basis of whichever particular focal question is being asked. Doing both then requires tailoring all supporting analyses accordingly.

4. Enhancing the goal also requires modifying one's concept of methodological success. We need to embrace additional, patient-centered success measures, such as those presented in section 2.2. These additional measures focus on individual patient predictive accuracy rather than on comparative factor potency.

5. The fundamental distinction between achieving comparative factor potency and achieving predictive accuracy at the individual patient level was made by Dr. Ware in his 2006 *New England Journal* article. Dr. Ware pointed out that achieving the former goal does not guarantee achieving the latter. PCM has been designed to bridge this gap.

6. Achieving the enhanced goal of predictive accuracy at the individual patient level requires making selective modifications to a number of analytical procedures. Examples of such modifications have been presented in sections 2.3 through 2.9.

PCM relies on four somewhat novel procedural devices whose combined impact is both cumulative and interactive. These four devices are as follows.

1. Analysis always begins with a focal question and a targeted patient. Some salient event or patient state or otherwise interesting end point is chosen at the outset. Analysis is uniformly focused on drawing predictive conclusions related to that question for a targeted, individual patient.

Altering the focal question can and typically does alter the appropriateness of various analytical procedures adopted to answer it. Altering even the way the focal question is phrased (e.g., the manner in which its answer is measured) may justify a completely different analysis. Altering the identity of the targeted patient can have the same effect.

Contrast this with current prognostic practice. Typically, a standard index is constructed for traditional or conventional factors, such as the AJCC T1/T2/T3/T4 index for primary tumor thickness in melanoma. That standard index is then applied uniformly to virtually all focal questions and to virtually all targeted patients.

2. Unless no candidate prognostic factors bear a systematic relationship to answering the focal question, selective stratification generally improves predictive accuracy.

Stratification means selecting one (or a small subset) of the candidate factors and using it (or them) as a means to stratify patients prior to using the remaining prognostic factors as inputs to (independent variables of) a prognostic model whose output (dependent variable) answers the focal question.

A detailed prognostic algorithm is generally incorporated within a prognostic model. Such is the case when a prognostic model is based on regression analysis or some other statistical procedure that estimates specific numeric parameters to fit the model to a sample of training data.

Which prognostic factors are appropriate candidates for stratification? Widely understood and routinely recorded factors related to disease progression are the appropriate candidates. Widely understood means traditional or conventional. This tends to lower resistance within the professional community to their systematic incorporation in all prognostic analyses. Routinely recorded guarantees that all prognostic analyses begin with observations that are already being made about most patients. No patients should be excluded from PCM simply because it cannot be determined in which population stratum they belong.

Among appropriate candidates the prognostic factor (or combination of factors) demonstrating the most potent predictive (causal or correlational) relationship with the focal question is frequently the best one (combination) to be used as a stratification variable. The stronger the relationship linking the stratification variable to the prediction being sought, the more likely will the separate strata so formed be internally homogeneous (in a predictive sense), even in the face of cross-stratum heterogeneity.

AJCC stage was chosen as the stratification variable for both melanoma patients and breast cancer patients. Stage of disease development is a well-documented and widely understood index, carefully constructed from potent prognostic factors. Staging is an integral part of most initial cancer diagnoses. These considerations made AJCC stage an appropriate candidate. It was then chosen from among the appropriate candidates because it was shown to possess the single most potent predictive impact in both cancers.

We are not claiming that stage of disease development is always the best stratification variable. The best variable is the one that has the most potent predictive impact relative to the focal question. Change the focal question, and the best stratification variable may well change with it. Thus, if the positive or negative outcome of a sentinel lymph node biopsy were the focal event to be predicted, stage of disease development would be less appropriate. Stage at diagnosis is an index that incorporates current nodal status as a component factor, yet early stages prior to nodal involvement might still be appropriate.

Stratification does require significantly larger sample sizes for statistical estimation. It also increases the risk of overfitting the algorithm to the particular observations used as training data.

By training data we mean all empirical data used to construct a prognostic algorithm useful in making individually tailored patient predictions.

3. Preprocessing prognostic factors prior to using them as inputs to (independent variables of) some form of regression analysis designed to answer the focal question frequently improves the efficacy of the regression. The Scale Partitioning and Spacing Algorithm (SPSA) described in sections 2.5, 2.6, and 2.7 implements preprocessing in PCM.

The concept of preprocessing raw data inputs to improve analytical efficacy is hardly novel. The AJCC and others have been doing this for many years. Patient age at diagnosis, anatomical site of primary tumor, and tumor thickness are all converted by the AJCC into standardized indexes in melanoma. AJCC stage combines T-scale, N-scale, and M-scale values (and other prognostic measurements) into a single, classificatory index in both melanoma and breast cancer.

SPSA is PCM's principal preprocessing procedure. SPSA is novel. It is fully automated in the form of a computerized algorithm. It is generally applicable to all prognostic factors. If applied to dichotomously defined factors (e.g., to patient sex), SPSA simply replicates, in effect, whatever standardized index may already exist. If applied to factors with more than two measured values, it creates a "shaped" standardized index (e.g., a UIRI). When applied to melanoma tumor thickness, SPSA's UIRI reproduces quite closely the AJCC's currently defined T1/T2/T3/T4 index (see Figure 3). However, when applied to melanoma mitotic rate, SPSA creates a novel, somewhat surprising, and highly suggestive UIRI (see Figure 4). It also creates UIRIs for newly discovered prognostic factors, such as biomarkers.

Besides these advantages, SPSA tailors its UIRIs, separately, both to each focal question being asked and to each separate population stratum containing patients similar to a targeted patient. Change the focal question or change the targeted patient, and SPSA will likely produce a different UIRI based on different cut points that generate different regression coefficients. Proceed beyond the factor-centered orientation and its implicit assumption of just one "proper," comprehensive patient population that all research efforts should seek to characterize. Then, separately tailored UIRIs become methodological improvements—not evidence of "biased" or "non-population-based" scholarship.

Sections 3 and 4 showed that such preprocessing by SPSA and the uniform substitution of corresponding UIRI indexes for each prognostic factor (originally calibrated in terms of its respective raw measurement scale) regularly improves the goodness of fit of the mathematical model underlying logistic regression. Appendix A illustrates goodness-of-fit improvement in the analysis of mitotic rate both by logistic regression and by Cox regression.

Substituting UIRI indexes also serves to normalize all regression inputs. UIRI values are always on the same measurement scale. Regression outputs indicating relative factor potency, such as relative risks (hazard ratios) in Cox regression, are thereby rendered comparable. Mere visual inspection suffices. One need not adjust one's interpretation of tabled output statistics for diversity among raw factor measurement scales.

Normalization also enables the proportional weighting procedure described in section 2.8 and an intuitively appealing way to compare the relative predictive potency of separate prognostic factors.

Scale partitioning and spacing via SPSA tend to improve predictive accuracy. This occurs both with and without stratification.

SPSA does require significantly larger sample sizes for statistical estimation. As with stratification, it therefore increases the risk of overfitting the prognostic algorithm to whatever empirical observations are used as training data.

4. The SPSA algorithm deals with missing observations of prognostic factors in an unusual manner. Exactly how is described in detail in sections 2.5, 2.6, and 2.7.

   A judgment is required to ensure that systematically different mechanisms underlying the absence of data are not improperly combined into a single category. It is analogous to the judgment required to combine different observation-censoring mechanisms into a single category in Kaplan-Meier and Cox regression analyses.

   Dealing with missing observations in the SPSA manner sometimes does and sometimes does not improve the goodness of fit of the logistic and Cox regression models.

   When combined with stratification, dealing with missing observations in the SPSA manner generally does improve the predictive accuracy of both logistic and Cox regression. In part, this is because default values assigned to patients with missing observations on some prognostic factor differ systematically according to the separate stratum each patient occupies. The more predictively potent the stratifying variable, the more discriminating the assigned, stratum-specific default values become.

   However, SPSA's special way of handling missing observations is not the sole mechanism of improvement. Parallel comparative analyses of PCM's other improvement devices were executed for both melanoma and breast cancer patients. Remarkably similar patterns of predictive improvement were realized in the two training samples from implementing PCM's other devices both with and without missing observations. The results of these two sensitivity analyses rule out attributing predictive improvement solely to SPSA's unusual handling of missing data.

Practicing physicians may find the following interpretation of PCM appealing.

1. Retain the current practice of using initial stage at diagnosis as the basis for probabilistic predictions of individual patient outcomes. AJCC stage stratifies patients according to their risk of experiencing numerous salient focal events. Survival probabilities, organized by initial stage and periodically published by the AJCC, remain as each patient's baseline prediction.
2. Then, modify each baseline prediction either upward or downward for an individual patient by applying the prediction algorithm derived from our proposed patient-centered methodology. Widespread access to a PCM-driven, Internet-based service center would be most helpful in this regard. Whatever prognostic factors are known about any patient may be entered into the prognostic algorithm to calculate the appropriate upward or downward adjustment.
3. Adjusted probabilities may then be used to guide individually tailored patient lifestyle choices, treatment selections, and other patient management decisions—such as undergoing specific diagnostic tests.
4. Relative factor potency weights assigned by PCM to a patient's AJCC stage may also be used in very much the same manner to decide which additional prognostic factor observations not yet obtained would be predictively useful to complete that patient's initial diagnosis.

Careful consideration of the overfitting issue is especially appropriate when stratification and preprocessing via SPSA are employed together. It then becomes essential to verify that apparent improvements in predictive accuracy are real—not spurious. Otherwise, applying PCM to training samples of small or intermediate size could be misleading.

What does statistical overfitting mean, and when does it become a serious prognostic problem?

A prognostic model is fitted via some statistical technique (regression analysis) to some particular collection of empirical observations. Empirical observations are made on selected attributes (prognostic factors) of selected entities (a training sample of patients). The statistical technique produces a prognostic algorithm. Inputs to (independent variables of) the algorithm are values of or indexes constructed from the observed attributes. The output (dependent variable) answers (probabilistically) the focal question.

The prognostic algorithm is fitted to a particular collection of empirical observations by choosing a specific set of (numeric) model parameters. The chosen parameters are those that render most plausible (e.g., most likely or prediction-error-minimizing) the observations actually contained in the training data if the assumed underlying model properly characterizes the entities and their related attributes in the population (stratum) from which that sample was obtained. Hence, training means statistical fitting of the parameters of a particular population model to a specific sample of observations. The prognostic algorithm is trained via the sample observations.

When the number of observations in a training sample becomes "too small" relative to the number of model parameters fitted to the observed data, the resulting prognostic algorithm is said to be overfitted. Its number of observations typically serves as a count of the number of degrees of freedom inherent in a training sample. The number of statistically independent observations in the sample is the dimensionality of (i.e., the number of orthogonal dimensions constituting) its sample space.

Sample sizes are frequently characterized as either "too small" or "large enough" by simple rules of thumb. An example would be that overfitting is avoided so long as the number of sample observations in the training data is at least ten times the number of parameters estimated by the fitted prognostic algorithm. Otherwise, the algorithm may be overfitted. This is because statistical estimation reduces the number of degrees of freedom remaining in the data. The estimation procedure uses them up. Apparent accuracy of estimation is improved at the expense of the degrees of freedom so consumed. We might think of degrees of freedom as the currency we must expend in order to purchase additional accuracy.

A hypothetical example in the spirit of our patient-centered methodology may help to clarify these concepts. The example illustrates how stratifying training data into successively more subsamples and constructing a separate prognostic algorithm for each separate subsample serves to increase apparent accuracy. It does so by consuming more and more degrees of freedom from the data. It also shows how the appearance of perfect accuracy can be achieved when all degrees of freedom are eventually used up, but how misleading such a spurious result becomes.

Suppose we wish to predict the magnitude of tumor growth on the basis of time elapsed since initial diagnosis. Imagine that:

1. a training sample of twenty cancer patients is collected;
2. pairs of observations are made on each patient's tumor mass, coupled with the time elapsed since diagnosis when that mass is observed; and
3. a simple linear function is fitted as a prognostic algorithm to the twenty pairs of sample observations via least-squares; such that
4. each patient's predicted mass may be calculated as some number (the first of two least-squares-estimated parameters, serving as the Y-intercept of the linear function), plus the time elapsed since diagnosis, multiplied by another number (the second of the two estimated parameters, serving as the slope of the linear prediction function); where
5. the estimated slope and intercept values would be called coefficients of regression if least-squares estimation were performed in the context of a simple linear regression analysis.

Unless the twenty observation pairs fall exactly along a straight line, there will be at least one difference between predicted and observed tumor masses. We can define the sum of these squared (or absolute) differences as the total prediction error.

Unless the fitted straight line is exactly horizontal (i.e., unless the second estimated slope parameter is exactly zero), suggesting absolutely no relationship linking tumor mass to elapsed time, the total prediction error will be reduced. Reduction, here, means reduction compared to ignoring all elapsed times and simply predicting that every patient's tumor mass will always be the mean of the twenty masses actually observed.

The linear prediction algorithm possesses two parameters defining its slope and intercept, respectively. It consumes two of the original twenty degrees of freedom. This minimally satisfies the illustrative rule of thumb. Overfitting is said to be avoided, since the sample size (twenty) is ten times the number of fitting parameters (two).

Now let us engage in a hypothetical procedure that will appear to improve predictive accuracy, even when no underlying relationship exists. That is, assume that the twenty observations are completely random and, therefore, that the best-fitting straight line is approximately horizontal (zero slope), and proceed as follows.

Imagine, first, that the sample is randomly divided into two subsamples of ten patients. Each subsample now contains ten pairs of the original observations. If two separate linear prediction algorithms are then fitted, respectively, to the two subsamples, the total prediction error (summed over both subsamples) will typically be slightly reduced. This is because the smaller size of each subsample permits a somewhat closer fit to its respective best-fitting straight line. It becomes somewhat easier to fit a single line to a smaller number of data points, even when the data are completely random. However, it costs four of the original twenty degrees of freedom to obtain this seeming improvement in predictive accuracy.

Imagine that the sample is again randomly divided, this time into five subsamples of four patients each. When five separate linear prediction algorithms are then fitted, respectively, to the five subsamples, this consumes ten of the original twenty degrees of freedom. The total prediction error will likely be further reduced, if only slightly, for the same reason.

The final step in this hypothetical process is to randomly subdivide the twenty patients into ten subsamples containing two patients each. Fitting ten separate linear prediction algorithms, respectively, to the ten subsamples consumes all of the original twenty degrees of freedom. It also reduces the total prediction error to zero. This is because each subsample contains only two data points (one for each patient), and a nonvertical straight line can be fitted exactly to any two successive (i.e., noncoincident) elapsed times.

There is a lesson here. Because there was no underlying relationship to begin with, the ten separately fitted straight lines will likely bear no relationship to one another. They will point in every which direction, reflecting the assumed nonrelationship. Yet the error of prediction seems to have been completely eliminated.

The lesson is that reducing prediction error (even to zero) does not, by itself, guarantee the existence of any such relationship. The cost in degrees of freedom used up must also be considered. If fitting the prognostic algorithm consumes "too many" degrees of freedom from the training data, the apparent improvement in predictive accuracy may be spurious. It may signify overfitting, rather than a true, underlying predictive relationship. Popular rules of thumb are designed to protect against this kind of threat.

PCM consumes many more degrees of freedom inherent within its training data than a typical, factor-centered analysis. Stratification, preprocessing via SPSA, and SPSA's manner of dealing with missing observations all involve the fitting of additional parameters—over and above the parameters that are subsequently fitted to training data via multiple regression analysis. That is why special care must be exercised to avoid overfitting.

Protection against overfitting is provided internally by the admissibility requirements described in section 2.5 and by the various procedures described in sections 2.6 and 2.7. Collectively, these are designed to support reasonably stable statistical estimates of predictive relationships shown by previous research to link selected prognostic factors to the focal question.

A far superior protection would be provided by thoroughly tested theory. If we knew with some confidence the exact nature of the biological mechanisms linking, for example, primary tumor size or the expression of various genes to salient patient outcomes, we would not need SPSA. We would understand in detail the nature of their predictive relationships. Empirically confirmed theory would supply both the shape and the magnitude of such relationships. Where SPSA is particularly useful is in the current situation. Many stable underlying biological relationships really do exist. Their direction of impact is generally known. However, we have yet to ascertain their detailed mechanics. We must still rely heavily on statistical models fitted to observational data to generate relationships that are predictively useful.

Sample size remains as a major issue. Our full-blown patient-centered methodology is not designed for small to intermediate-sized training samples. To achieve nonspurious improvements in predictive accuracy requires sample sizes at least in the thousands—preferably tens of thousands. This assumes, of course, the existence of nonspurious indicators to serve as prognostic factors. Otherwise, merely increasing sample size will not help.

It was just because both the melanoma and breast cancer training samples contained little more than a thousand patients each that stratification into only three risk subgroups occurred. Larger training sample sizes would have permitted stratification into a greater number of risk subgroups. Ideally, training sample sizes would be sufficiently large to permit stratification into at least as many distinct risk subgroups as there are statistically distinguishable stages of disease progression identified by the AJCC.

It is fortunate that some of PCM's analytical devices can still be applied to intermediate-sized training samples (e.g., to samples containing only hundreds of patients). Using SPSA to preprocess prognostic factor inputs to a logistic or a Cox regression generally improves the goodness of fit of the assumed underlying model. If the regression involves only a few prognostic factors as independent variables, improved predictive accuracy can also be achieved, without risking excessive overfitting. Both benefits were illustrated in appendix A.

There is also the follow-up issue. Merely having a lot of observational data is not enough. Our melanoma sample spanned more than thirty-nine years. Our breast cancer sample spanned more than fifty-one years. Since the methodology is designed to make prognoses of progressive diseases and because it seeks to tailor these prognoses to the complete range of individual patients, follow-up periods comparable in duration to the disease's gestation and development times are required.

Data quality is another critical consideration. Our patient-centered methodology employs a number of reasonably sophisticated analytical techniques. It does more than just summarize data in terms of means, standard deviations, and cross-tabulations. Noisy patient data, containing many incorrect and inconsistent observations, can neutralize the efficacy of these otherwise useful techniques. Typically, the more sophisticated the analysis, the more easily it can be compromised by even a little noise in the data.

We must acknowledge that our two illustrative training samples contained data of distinctly higher-than-average quality. That is an important part of the reason they were chosen. Medical records for the 1,222 melanoma patients were checked, rechecked, and selectively corrected many times during the last decade at UCSF. When initially received from Finland in 1999, the 1,225-patient breast cancer data set was unusually complete and free of inconsistencies. We do not claim that our patient-centered methodology would perform as well on the less clean medical records commonly encountered throughout the world. Much existing medical data would require thorough "precleaning" before it could be usefully exploited by PCM.

The patient-centered orientation has been characterized as an extension of the more traditional factor-centered orientation. It rests upon successful prior discovery of genuine prognostic connections. For example, prognostic factors are inadmissible to PCM unless or until both the existence and direction of their impact upon a specified focal event has already been established for patients similar to a targeted patient. Establishing such connections is a factor-centered enterprise.

In view of this close relationship, are the various devices employed by PCM to improve individually tailored predictive accuracy always appropriate for drawing traditional factor-centered conclusions? The answer is no. Some of these devices may sometimes be appropriate, but not all of them are always appropriate.

A clear counterexample may be instructive.

Imagine an exploratory research context in which the impact, if any, of a previously unfamiliar biomarker on the progress of a particular cancer is under study. The existence, direction, and magnitude of such a linkage are obvious targets of investigation. An appropriate null hypothesis would be the complete absence of any linkage.

Would it then be proper:

1. to gather a sample of observations that might indicate a linkage;
2. to check the sample data for any apparent direction of impact by performing a cross-tabulation or by calculating a sample correlation coefficient or by doing something similar;
3. to formulate, accordingly, the sample-data-indicated directional alternate hypothesis; and
4. to perform, therefore, a one-tail statistical test of the null hypothesis?

The norms of classical hypothesis testing forbid such a procedure. In general, it is not proper to utilize any observed aspects of sample data to formulate null and alternate hypotheses about the population from which the sample was obtained. Only null and alternate hypotheses formulated without reference to observed sample data are properly testable by such data.

A good way to remain consistent with appropriate procedure is to formulate research hypotheses before gathering a sample. In an exploratory context, there is little basis for formulating anything other than a nondirectional alternate hypothesis. This calls for a two-tail test, not a one-tail test of the null hypothesis.

According to the same general principle, SPSA should not be applied to observed sample data in a classical hypothesis-testing context. If the goal of the analysis is to draw a factor-centered conclusion about the impact of some prognostic indicator on some salient focal event in some interesting population, first converting raw measurement data into a corresponding UIRI would be inappropriate. Using SPSA to construct a UIRI that optimally captures whatever underlying relationship appears to exist between the indicator and the focal event, and then using that same UIRI to test the null hypothesis that no such relationship exists is a clear violation of classical norms.

Constructing a UIRI is based on the assumption that an underlying relationship does exist in the population. Using a UIRI then to test whether or not such a relationship really exists constitutes circular and, therefore, inappropriate deductive reasoning. SPSA-generated UIRIs should not be so used in a traditional, factor-centered context. One must adopt a patient-centered orientation and its different goal to avoid circular reasoning.

Dr. Ware pointed out that achieving statistical significance (a factor-centered conclusion) does not guarantee achieving accurate, individually tailored predictions (the overarching patient-centered goal). We are acknowledging the reverse. What one does to improve the accuracy of individually tailored patient predictions is not necessarily appropriate in a factor-centered context.

We hope that the results reported herein will encourage some centralized organization with significant resources to replicate, if possible, the improvements in predictive accuracy that our patient-centered methodology appears to offer. This means selecting a particular progressive disease, such as a specific cancer, and launching a replication project. It is not unlike the situation where promising results have been achieved in phase I and phase II clinical trials and the next step is to achieve definitive results in phase III.

A replication project would entail:

1. obtaining a comprehensive, multi-institutional sample containing many thousand patients diagnosed with some particular disease;
2. gleaning from patient records data on selected focal events related to disease progression and a set of candidate prognostic factors known to be associated with each focal event;
3. thoroughly "precleaning" the collected data;
4. randomly partitioning the sample into a many-thousand-patient training subsample and a many-thousand-patient validation subsample;
5. fitting, first via traditional prognostic methodologies and then via PCM, separate prediction algorithms to the same training subsample;
6. applying each of the separate prediction algorithms to the validation subsample; and
7. finally, assessing the comparative predictive accuracy achieved by each separate algorithm when applied to the validation subsample.

If PCM produces significantly greater predictive accuracy in the validation subsample, then with a sufficiently large number of patients, such improvement cannot be attributed simply to overfitting its prediction algorithm to the training data.

Even better, this validation procedure mimics quite closely the anticipated practical application of PCM. Some institution could produce and continually update prediction algorithms relating to selected focal events and stratified by differential risk of disease progression. Individually tailored event predictions could then be produced and delivered via the Internet to new patients and their doctors. A new patient is one not involved in producing and updating the prediction algorithms.

The ability to incorporate nontraditional and nonconventional prognostic factors (e.g., newly discovered biomarkers) into PCM has always been one of its major design objectives. However, incorporating additional prognostic factors also increases the risk of overfitting. This is one reason why convincing replication requires such large sample sizes. Another reason is to be comprehensive enough to enable predictions for statistically infrequent focal events and for patients dwelling in sparsely inhabited population strata.

Our principal recommendation is that at least one large-scale replication project be undertaken that focuses on a specific progressive disease (cancer).

Have we demonstrated sufficient proof of concept to justify this recommendation? We believe that we have.

Appendix F describes two limited-scope, split-sample reliability analyses designed to validate PCM's apparently superior predictive accuracy in just the manner described above. To eliminate the risk of overfitting, the scope of these analyses was limited to include only the six AJCC traditional prognostic factors in melanoma and the corresponding five conventional factors used to predict breast cancer.

Our 1,222 melanoma patients were randomly partitioned into a training subsample of 800 and a validation subsample of 422. Similarly, our 1,225 breast cancer patients were randomly partitioned into a training subsample of 800 and a validation subsample of 425. The procedures outlined in section 3 and section 4 were then applied, respectively, to the two training subsamples of 800 patients each.

The goal of the split-sample analyses was to reproduce in the two 800-patient training subsamples PCM's superior predictive accuracy, as reported in sections 3 and 4 for the two complete samples, and then to use prediction algorithms produced from the training subsamples to replicate PCM's superior predictive accuracy in both validation subsamples. That goal was achieved. The tables presented in appendix F document these results.

Highlights from appendix F are as follows.

1. The traditional factor-centered base case prediction algorithm produced from the 800-patient melanoma training subsample via standard logistic regression analysis was applied to the 422 patients in the validation subsample. This produced 422 individually tailored MM DEATH probabilities with an estimated AUC of 0.7747.
2. The practice-centered base case prediction algorithm produced from the same melanoma training subsample via dummy-variable logistic regression analysis solely on the basis of AJCC stage at initial diagnosis was also applied to patients in the validation subsample. This produced a second set of 422 MM DEATH probabilities with an estimated AUC of 0.7902.
3. This improvement in AUC was accompanied by an index of error reduction = 0.2464 and a normalized Wilcoxon Z statistic = 4.27, with a two-tail p value < 0.00005.
4. The prediction algorithm produced from the same six traditional prognostic factor observations made on the same 800-patient melanoma training subsample via our PCM methodology was also applied to the 422 patients in the validation subsample. This produced a third set of 422 MM DEATH probabilities with an estimated AUC of 0.7980.
5. Compared to the factor-centered base case analysis, the PCM improvement in AUC generated an index of error reduction = 0.4123 and a normalized Wilcoxon Z statistic = 6.29, with a two-tail p value < 0.00005.
6. Compared to the practice-centered base case analysis, the PCM improvement in AUC was accompanied by an index of error reduction = 0.1943 and a normalized Wilcoxon Z statistic = 2.73, with a two-tail p value 0.0063.
7. The conventional factor-centered base case prediction algorithm produced from the 800-patient breast cancer training subsample via standard logistic regression analysis was applied to the 425 patients in the validation subsample. This produced 425 individually tailored MBC DEATH probabilities with an estimated AUC of 0.7631.
8. The practice-centered base case prediction algorithm produced from the same breast cancer training subsample via dummy-variable logistic

regression analysis solely on the basis of AJCC stage at initial diagnosis was also applied to patients in the validation subsample. This produced a second set of 425 MBC DEATH probabilities with an estimated AUC of 0.8212.

9. This improvement in AUC was accompanied by an index of error reduction = 0.3600 and a normalized Wilcoxon Z statistic = 6.22, with a two-tail p value < 0.00005.

10. The prediction algorithm produced from the same five conventional prognostic factor observations made on the same 800-patient breast cancer training subsample via our PCM methodology was also applied to the 425 patients in the validation subsample. This produced a third set of 425 MBC DEATH probabilities with an estimated AUC of 0.8785.

11. Compared to the factor-centered base case analysis, the PCM improvement in AUC was accompanied by an index of error reduction = 0.5953 and a normalized Wilcoxon Z statistic = 11.20, with a two-tail p value < 0.00005.

12. Compared to the practice-centered base case analysis, the PCM improvement in AUC was accompanied by an index of error reduction = 0.3082 and a normalized Wilcoxon Z statistic = 6.36, with a two-tail p value < 0.00005.

13. Strikingly, none of these highly significant improvements in predictive accuracy for either melanoma or breast cancer resulted from adding more prognostic factors to the analyses. All improvements were achieved simply by substituting PCM's novel procedural devices for the standard methods used to analyze traditional and conventional prognostic factors.

14. All of these improvements were derived from analysis of the two validation subsamples. Prediction algorithms were obtained, respectively, from the two training subsamples and then applied to the validation subsamples. Since each training subsample was completely distinct from its corresponding validation subsample, none of these improvements can be attributed to overfitting the specific training data. There had to exist stable underlying relationships linking traditional and conventional prognostic factors to five-year disease-specific death to support such predictive improvements in the validation subsamples.

Such replicated predictive improvements are most encouraging, but not definitive. Something akin to a phase III clinical trial has yet to be performed. The recommended replication project based on a larger and more comprehensive sample of patients than the two data sets that were available to us to achieve proof of concept is still required.

If replicated, a sizable long-term investment might also be justified to exploit PCM's benefits. Significant resources would then be required:

1. to obtain a large number of medical records from many different institutional and other sources;

2. to purge enough errors and inconsistencies from these records to support the sometimes sophisticated analyses inherent in PCM;

3. to update and maintain these records over a sufficiently long time period to satisfy follow-up requirements;

4. to establish and maintain an analysis system that may be continually enhanced with new and updated patient data;

5. to use this analysis system to deliver tailored individual prognoses to physicians and to their patients on demand (e.g., via a permanent, Internet-based service center);

6. to extend the reach of this system by funding on a continuing basis the search for new, nontraditional prognostic factors;

7. to signal that this is intended to be a continuing and ongoing effort in many other ways, too, and to actually facilitate that result; and
8. to provide effective incentives that will induce various institutional and noninstitutional players to continue to participate in and cooperate with this effort on an ongoing basis.

It goes without saying that these significant resources must also be committed over a long time period.

This is a time in history when many relevant budgets are shrinking. Since making a significant long-term investment requires a successful large-scale replication of PCM's improved prognostic accuracy, we should close by underscoring the likely immediacy of benefits, should definitive replication be achieved.

The two limited-scope, split-sample reliability analyses strongly suggest that an appreciable share of PCM's total increase in predictive accuracy can be realized quickly, easily, and inexpensively. Just alter the way traditional and conventional prognostic risk factors are currently being analyzed. Incorporate PCM's novel procedural devices into the analysis whenever the goal is to make accurate, individually tailored patient predictions—assuming that sample sizes are adequate.

This simple alteration accounted for close to half of the total improvement (measured in AUC gain) over the practice-centered base case realized by our complete sample of 1,222 melanoma patients. It accounted for more than three quarters of the total improvement (also measured in AUC gain) over the practice-centered base case realized by our complete sample of 1,225 breast cancer patients.

Yes, ongoing research to identify additional, nontraditional prognostic factors is definitely in order. No, we need not wait until that ongoing research achieves fruition. Substantial benefit seems immediately realizable at far less cost. Doing so might demonstrate quite dramatically how we can allocate our limited resources more wisely.

Appendix A

A Simplified Illustration and Assessment of the Patient-Centered Methodology

Disease-specific death within five years of diagnosis is predicted on the basis
of mitotic rate (MITRATE) within the primary tumor. Analyses are based on our
training sample of 1,222 melanoma patients. The focal event is MM DEATH=<5YRS.
MM signifies metastatic melanoma. Its complementary event is labeled DSS>5YRS.
DSS signifies disease-specific survival. Summary statistics for MITRATE and the
focal event are shown below. "*" signifies undefined (missing) observations.
****

SUMMARY STATISTICS	ATTRIBUTE MITRATE	
n DEFINED	944	The MITRATE attribute counts the number of mitoses observed in a high-powered microscopic field (hpf) of one square millimeter.
MINIMUM	0	
MEDIAN	3	
MAXIMUM	22	
MEAN	4.2044	
STD. DEV.	3.6542	

VALUE OF ATTRIBUTE MITRATE	ABSOLUTE FREQUENCIES (COUNTS)	RELATIVE FREQUENCIES (PROPORTIONS)	CUMULATIVE RELATIVE FREQUENCIES
0	74	.0606	.0606
1	160	.1309	.1915
2	145	.1187	.3101
3	111	.0908	.4010
4	96	.0786	.4795
5	119	.0974	.5769
6	26	.0213	.5982
7	56	.0458	.6440
8	71	.0581	.7021
9	11	.0090	.7111
10	21	.0172	.7283
11	1	.0008	.7291
12	26	.0213	.7504
13	2	.0016	.7520
14	2	.0016	.7537
15	5	.0041	.7578
16	3	.0025	.7602
18	12	.0098	.7700
22	3	.0025	.7725
*	278	.2275	1.0000
TOTAL	1222	1.0000	

VALUE OF ATTRIBUTE DSS5YR	ABSOLUTE FREQUENCIES (COUNTS)	RELATIVE FREQUENCIES (PROPORTIONS)	CUMULATIVE RELATIVE FREQUENCIES
DSS>5YRS	941	.7700	.7700
MM DEATH=<5YRS	281	.2300	1.0000
TOTAL	1222	1.0000	

****

The partitioning procedure outlined in section 2.6 is executed on the raw measurement scale of MITRATE. The command procedure performing the partitioning and rescaling is called SPSA. It implements the Scale Partitioning and Spacing Algorithm. Just as presented on the previous page, literal computer output will be enclosed between two horizontal strings of asterisks.

Notice from the computer printout on the next few pages six useful features of the SPSA command.

1. The first two input expressions identify, respectively, the focal event to be predicted (embodied in the DSS5YR attribute) and the prognostic indicator (the MITRATE attribute) whose raw measurement scale is to be partitioned and "spaced" so as to provide as accurate an individually tailored probabilistic prediction of the focal event as possible.

   Both expressions may be entered either as already-defined patient attributes (as illustrated in this example) or as mathematical functions, indexes, and so forth, modifying or combining already-defined attributes.

2. The third input expression establishes the minimum partition (subscale) size for the SPSA algorithm. Although typically twenty-five patients, in this example it is seventy-five patients.

3. The fourth and fifth input expressions indicate that the UIRI produced by the SPSA command is to be submitted, automatically, to a Cox regression analysis whose first two inputs are logically related to the first input of the SPSA command.

   The first input of the SPSA command identifies the focal event to be predicted in probabilistic terms. The first two inputs of the automatically invoked COXREG command define the time elapsed between some reference event (e.g., initial diagnosis) and the occurrence of that focal event (e.g., disease-specific death). The fourth and fifth inputs of the SPSA command are passed through as the first two inputs of the corresponding COXREG command.

   The patient-centered output of a logistic regression is an individually tailored focal event probability (a separate probability for each patient). The patient-centered output of the corresponding Cox regression performed on the same data is an individually tailored survival function describing also in probabilistic terms how long that same patient will survive without experiencing the focal event.

   An automatic Cox regression is optional. It only occurs when these two additional inputs appear at the end of the SPSA command line. When executed, the automatic option performs a dummy-variable Cox regression, where 0/1 dummy variables are defined to reflect the optimal partitioning of the indicator's raw measurement scale determined by SPSA. The operational definitions of these one or more 0/1 dummy variables are transmitted as additional parameters to the COXREG command. Missing or otherwise undefined values of the prognostic indicator are not permitted with this automatic option.

   The automatic option is quite helpful in deciding via trial and error how large to set the minimum partition size for SPSA. The minimum size can be increased just enough by this look-ahead feature both to ensure that the relative risks generated by the corresponding Cox regression are in the same rank order as the UIRI probabilities generated by SPSA and to obtain p values on all 0/1 dummy variables in the Cox regression "small enough" to corroborate a genuine monotonic impact.

A trial-and-error procedure was executed in the example shown on the next few pages to determine the minimum partition size of seventy-five patients. It illustrates one of the internal mechanisms within SPSA to deal with potential overfitting of the prognostic algorithm to the training data.

4. Optionally, a scatterplot may be produced for any UIRI. It provides a visual representation of the "shape" of the relationship linking a candidate indicator to the focal event it is attempting to predict. An enhanced scatterplot was displayed in Figure 4 of section 3.3.

5. Although not exercised in the example, there is an additional option to weight unequally the sensitivity and specificity achieved by SPSA's partitioning procedure. Some research or practical contexts might suggest unequal weighting.

6. All command procedures may be set to generate written output in extensively annotated format. Displayed results are explained and interpreted in substantial detail. Such is the case with the following output.

* *

Standard ASCII string expression number 1 is just the attribute DSS5YR.
Numeric expression number 2 is just the attribute MITRATE.
Numeric expression number 3 is 75.
Numeric expression number 4 is DATEINT(DATEDIAG,DATEDIED) IF CAUSEOFD= "MELANOSIS" OR CAUSEOFD="METASTATIC MELANOMA".
Numeric expression number 5 is DATEINT(DATEDIAG,DATELDSS).

The effective working data set contains the subset of 944 PATIENTs selected by the IF-defined antecedent condition MITRATE#UNDEFN from the DSSPROG WDS in the context DEC10.

The first two expressions (parameters) in the command specification are completely defined on 944 PATIENTs. The first expression is defined, while the second is undefined on 0 PATIENTs. The 944 PATIENTs whose first value is defined and whose second value may or may not be defined constitute the effective sample of all analyses performed by the SPSA command.

2 distinct values of the first expression in the command specification and 19 distinct values of the second expression are defined for the effective sample.

Analysis will focus on the state or event identified as MM DEATH=<5YRS. The alternative state or event is identified as DSS>5YRS. Sample 2, containing 232 PATIENTs, is in the focal MM DEATH=<5YRS category, while sample 1, containing 712 PATIENTs, is in the alternative DSS>5YRS category.

In order to qualify as a directionally admissible indicator expression for predictive purposes, sample 1 values of the second expression cannot be systematically larger, in a rank-order sense, than its sample 2 values. A Mann-Whitney test has verified that sample 1 values are systematically *SMALLER*, with a one-tail p value of .0000. Taking note of this test result, the analysis will proceed.

PROVISIONAL INDICATOR CUT OFF VALUE	SPECIFICITY PROPORTION	SENSITIVITY PROPORTION	WEIGHTED AVERAGE PROPORTION
1	.0969	.9784	.5377
2	.3034	.9224	.6129
3	.4747	.8233	.6490
4	.6124	.7672	.6898
5	.7121	.6595	.6858
6	.8146	.4612	.6379
7	.8441	.4397	.6419
8	.8890	.3362	.6126
9	.9396	.1853	.5625
10	.9466	.1595	.5531
11	.9635	.1207	.5421
12	.9649	.1207	.5428
13	.9817	.0603	.5210
14	.9846	.0603	.5224
15	.9860	.0560	.5210
16	.9888	.0431	.5159
18	.9888	.0302	.5095
22	.9958	.0000	.4979

The optimal cut off value of the indicator expression is 4. It is optimal in the sense that it maximizes the weighted average of the sensitivity and the specificity proportions achieved by the prediction. When their value of MITRATE is at least 4, PATIENTs are predicted to be in the MM DEATH=<5YRS category. When their value of MITRATE is less than 4, PATIENTs are predicted to be in the DSS>5YRS category. Using this binary cut off, the weighted average of the sensitivity and the specificity proportions is raised to a maximum of .6898. The weight applied to the sensitivity proportion in calculating the weighted average is .5000. When the weight is exactly .5000 (i.e., when the weighted average is nothing more than a simple average), the same cut off value is also optimal in the sense that it maximizes the estimated area under a ROC curve formed from just a binary cut off.

The second expression MITRATE qualifies as an admissible indicator of the first expression DSS5YR. The first expression simply distinguishes the focal from the alternative states or events. The SPSA command finds the most potent way to partition the indicator's raw measurement scale so as to maximize this discrimination on a univariate basis. It produces a Univariate Impact-Reflecting Index (UIRI). The UIRI may be substituted for the original indicator (second expression in the command specification) to improve predictive accuracy (e.g., in a logistic or Cox regression).

The indicator's optimal scale partitioning and numeric rescaling are embodied in the Univariate Impact-Reflecting Index (UIRI) produced by the Scale Partitioning and Spacing Algorithm (SPSA) with a minimum partition (subscale) size set equal to 75. The UIRI's operational definition is shown below.

```
18/234 IF MITRATE<2 ELSE
36/256 IF MITRATE>=2 AND MITRATE<4 ELSE
25/96 IF MITRATE=4 ELSE
51/145 IF MITRATE>=5 AND MITRATE<7 ELSE
59/127 IF MITRATE>=7 AND MITRATE<9 ELSE
43/86 IF MITRATE>=9
```

A file named UIRI_SCATTERPLOT.TXT has been created in the [DOSFILES] directory. It contains two columns of data. The first column is labeled UIRI and contains

UIRI values calculated for successive scale partitions of the second (indicator) expression in the SPSA command line. The second column is labeled with the operational definition of the second (indicator) expression itself to identify what is being plotted. The means of the indicator expression values in each successive partition are laid out along the horizontal X-axis of the scatterplot, and the corresponding UIRI values are laid out along the vertical Y-axis.

The effective working data set contains the subset of 944 PATIENTs selected by the IF-defined antecedent condition MITRATE#UNDEFN from the DSSPROG WDS in the context DEC10.

The effective sample size is 944. This means that the number of PATIENTs contained within the effective WDS whose elapsed focal event or censored times are all strictly positive and all of whose independent variables possess defined values is 944. The number of PATIENTs in the effective sample who experience the focal event is 328.

RESULTS OF COX REGRESSION ANALYSIS (PROPORTIONAL HAZARDS MODEL)

The dependent variable is either the time elapsed until the focal event occurs (focal event time), if the focal event does occur, or the time elapsed without the occurrence of the focal event (censored time), if the focal event has not yet occurred as of the latest observation. The dependent variable is embodied in the first two expressions (parameters) of the COXREG command shown below.

The first expression is DATEINT(DATEDIAG,DATEDIED) IF CAUSEOFD="MELANOSIS" OR CAUSEOFD="METASTATIC MELANOMA".
The second expression is DATEINT(DATEDIAG,DATELDSS).

The independent variable EXPRESSION3 is 1 IF MITRATE>=2 AND MITRATE<4 ELSE 0.
The independent variable EXPRESSION4 is 1 IF MITRATE=4 ELSE 0.
The independent variable EXPRESSION5 is 1 IF MITRATE>=5 AND MITRATE<7 ELSE 0.
The independent variable EXPRESSION6 is 1 IF MITRATE>=7 AND MITRATE<9 ELSE 0.
The independent variable EXPRESSION7 is 1 IF MITRATE>=9 ELSE 0.

Likelihood ratio chi-square statistic: 96.219, two-tail p value: .0000.
Score chi-square statistic: 101.530, two-tail p value: .0000.
Wald chi-square statistic: 90.659, two-tail p value: .0000.

All three chi-square statistics are based on 5 degrees of freedom and 944 observations, encompassing 308 distinct focal event times.

INDEPENDENT VARIABLE	REGRESSION COEFFICIENT	STANDARD DEVIATION	CHI-SQUARE (DF = 1)	2-TAIL P VALUE	RELATIVE RISK
EXPRESSION3	.4688	.1957	5.7369	.0166	1.5981
EXPRESSION4	.9726	.2240	18.8509	.0000	2.6449
EXPRESSION5	1.1048	.2000	30.5188	.0000	3.0185
EXPRESSION6	1.4662	.1960	55.9764	.0000	4.3329
EXPRESSION7	1.5520	.2117	53.7721	.0000	4.7210

VALUE OF PARTITIONED MITRATE SCALE	VALUE OF ATTRIBUTE DSS5YR		
	DSS>5YRS	MM DEATH=<5YRS	TOTAL
MITOTIC RATE 0 OR 1 per hpf	216	18	234
MITOTIC RATE 2 OR 3 per hpf	220	36	256
MITOTIC RATE 4 per hpf	71	25	96
MITOTIC RATE 5 OR 6 per hpf	94	51	145
MITOTIC RATE 7 OR 8 per hpf	68	59	127
MITOTIC RATE AT LEAST 9 per hpf	43	43	86
MITOTIC RATE UNDEFINED	229	49	278
TOTAL	941	281	1222

****

UIRI stands for Univariate Impact-Reflecting Index. For each subscale in the partitioned MITRATE scale the UIRI is set equal to the incidence (relative frequency) of the focal event (MM DEATH=<5YRS) among all patients falling into that subscale. Subscale relative frequencies are the likelihood-maximizing estimates of individual patient probabilities that result from a zero-one (0/1) dummy-variable logistic regression analysis. The resulting attribute is labeled LOGUIRI. This implements the procedure outlined in section 2.7.

Note that an extra scale partition has been added to the definition of the LOGUIRI attribute to account for the 278 missing or undefined values of mitotic rate. Note also that the LOGUIRI value (subscale relative frequency) associated with undefined observations (MITRATE=UNDEFN) falls well within the LOGUIRI distribution. In fact it falls approximately at the middle of the distribution. This is consistent with the presumption that missing observations are drawn from a subpopulation distributionally similar to the subpopulation from which defined observations are drawn. There is no apparent reason to interpret missing observations as signifying anything systematically unusual. They are just missing.

However, when the relative frequency of the focal event assigned to missing or undefined observations falls at either extreme of the UIRI distribution, this may signify something quite interesting. It suggests that these nonobservations may have been drawn from a systematically different subpopulation. It might well prove worthwhile to investigate further.

For example, the relative frequency of disease-specific death (UIRI value) assigned to missing observations of the anatomical location of a primary tumor in melanoma is often higher than the relative frequency (UIRI value) assigned to all known locations. This is because a missing observation may well indicate an unknown primary tumor. Patients with unknown primaries are often diagnosed at a later stage of disease development than patients with known primaries. Thus, in this instance, a missing observation can possess systematic predictive value.

****

DEFINE LOGUIRI:
18/234 IF MITRATE<2 ELSE
36/256 IF MITRATE>=2 AND MITRATE<4 ELSE
25/96 IF MITRATE=4 ELSE
51/145 IF MITRATE>=5 AND MITRATE<7 ELSE
59/127 IF MITRATE>=7 AND MITRATE<9 ELSE
43/86 IF MITRATE>=9 ELSE
49/278 IF MITRATE=UNDEFN

VALUE OF PARTITIONED MITRATE SCALE	VALUE OF ATTRIBUTE LOGUIRI							
	.0769	.1406	.1763	.2604	.3517	.4646	.5000	TOTAL
MITOTIC RATE 0 OR 1 per hpf	234	0	0	0	0	0	0	234
MITOTIC RATE 2 OR 3 per hpf	0	256	0	0	0	0	0	256
MITOTIC RATE UNDEFINED	0	0	278	0	0	0	0	278
MITOTIC RATE 4 per hpf	0	0	0	96	0	0	0	96
MITOTIC RATE 5 OR 6 per hpf	0	0	0	0	145	0	0	145
MITOTIC RATE 7 OR 8 per hpf	0	0	0	0	0	127	0	127
MITOTIC RATE AT LEAST 9 per hpf	0	0	0	0	0	0	86	86
TOTAL	234	256	278	96	145	127	86	1222

```
**********************************************************************
```

A chi-square test is performed on the cross-tabulation of LOGUIRI (the partitioned MITRATE scale) and the focal event. The calculated p value is quite small, suggesting a definite impact of MITRATE on MM DEATH=<5YRS. However, as was pointed out in section 5, this should not be interpreted as a classical hypothesis test in a factor-centered context. MITRATE has first been converted by SPSA into LOGUIRI, and chi-square is then computed from LOGUIRI values.

A highly suggestive unidirectional pattern is reflected in the conditional relative frequencies. Lower values of LOGUIRI are associated with DSS>5YRS. Higher values of LOGUIRI are associated with MM DEATH=<5YRS. This verifies the usual pattern repeatedly reported in the literature.

```
**********************************************************************
```

TABLE OF JOINT ABSOLUTE FREQUENCIES (COUNTS)

VALUE OF ATTRIBUTE LOGUIRI	VALUE OF ATTRIBUTE DSS5YR		
	DSS>5YRS	MM DEATH=<5YRS	TOTAL
.0769	216	18	234
.1406	220	36	256
.1763	229	49	278
.2604	71	25	96
.3517	94	51	145
.4646	68	59	127
.5000	43	43	86
TOTAL	941	281	1222

TABLE OF RELATIVE FREQUENCIES (PROPORTIONS) CONDITIONAL BY ROW

VALUE OF ATTRIBUTE LOGUIRI	VALUE OF ATTRIBUTE DSS5YR		
	DSS>5YRS	MM DEATH=<5YRS	TOTAL
.0769	.9231	.0769	1.0000
.1406	.8594	.1406	1.0000
.1763	.8237	.1763	1.0000
.2604	.7396	.2604	1.0000
.3517	.6483	.3517	1.0000
.4646	.5354	.4646	1.0000
.5000	.5000	.5000	1.0000

A chi-square statistical test was performed on the joint absolute frequencies.

The value of the chi-square statistic calculated for this table is 134.55, with 6 degree(s) of freedom.

The null hypothesis tested is that in the population, the attribute or expression whose 7 possible values are laid out along the rows of the table is *COMPLETELY UNRELATED* to (i.e., is distributed *STATISTICALLY INDEPENDENTLY* of) the attribute or expression whose 2 possible values are laid out along its columns.

Since there are more than two rows and/or more than two columns in the table, the alternate hypothesis must be nondirectional.

If the null hypothesis were true, the probability of generating a table at least as unfavorable to the null hypothesis as the above table in any direction would be .0000.

****
Separate logistic regression analyses are now performed, first on MITRATE (in its raw data form), and then on LOGUIRI, the impact-reflecting index produced by applying the SPSA command to MITRATE. In both analyses, the dependent variable is DSSDUMMY (a 0/1 version of the focal event, where DSS>5YRS is coded as 0, and MM DEATH=<5YRS is coded as 1).

Note how poorly the logistic regression model fits MITRATE in the first analysis. The reasonable-fit null hypothesis underlying both goodness-of-fit tests can be rejected at $p < 0.00005$. This casts doubt on the otherwise impressive logistic regression test results.

Note the improved results obtained in the second analysis from partitioning and "spacing" raw measurement values in the MITRATE scale to produce LOGUIRI. Both goodness-of-statistical-fit statistics now suggest a reasonable fit of the logistic regression model with the impact-reflecting index numbers. Also, the chi-square value assigned to the LOGUIRI regression coefficient is noticeably higher than the chi-square value assigned to the raw data MITRATE coefficient. This illustrates the additional benefit gained from preprocessing MITRATE via SPSA to produce LOGUIRI (but recall the classical hypothesis testing caveat).
****

Numeric expression number 1 is just the attribute DSSDUMMY.
Numeric expression number 2 is just the attribute MITRATE.

The effective working data set contains the 1222 PATIENTs constituting the DSSPROG WDS in the context DEC10.

After removing all undefined values from all expressions, the resulting number of PATIENTs for which each of the two expressions possesses a defined value is reduced to 944. This constitutes the effective sample size.

RESULTS OF LOGISTIC REGRESSION ANALYSIS (LINEAR MODEL)

The dependent variable is a binary-coded numeric variable whose values are either 0 or 1. It is embodied in the first expression (parameter) of the LOGREG command, which is just the attribute DSSDUMMY.

The independent variable MITRATE is just the attribute MITRATE.

Likelihood ratio chi-square statistic: 89.791, two-tail p value: .0000 (based on 1 degree of freedom and 944 complete observations).

INDEPENDENT VARIABLE	REGRESSION COEFFICIENT	STANDARD DEVIATION	CHI-SQUARE (DF = 1)	2-TAIL P VALUE	ODDS RATIO MULTIPLIER
intercept	-2.0245	.1346	226.1593	.0000	.1321
MITRATE	.1929	.0219	77.7168	.0000	1.2128

GOODNESS OF STATISTICAL FIT OF LOGISTIC REGRESSION MODEL

Pearson chi-square fit statistic (based on 17 degrees of freedom): 66.724, p value: .0000.

Deviance chi-square fit statistic (based on 17 degrees of freedom): 54.437, p value: .0000.

Numeric expression number 1 is just the attribute DSSDUMMY.
Numeric expression number 2 is just the attribute LOGUIRI.

The effective working data set contains the 1222 PATIENTs constituting the DSSPROG WDS in the context DEC10.

After removing all undefined values from all expressions the resulting number of PATIENTs for which each of the two expressions possesses a defined value is reduced to 1222. This constitutes the effective sample size.

RESULTS OF LOGISTIC REGRESSION ANALYSIS (LINEAR MODEL)

The dependent variable is a binary-coded numeric variable whose values are either 0 or 1. It is embodied in the first expression (parameter) of the LOGREG command, which is just the attribute DSSDUMMY.

The independent variable LOGUIRI is just the attribute LOGUIRI.

Likelihood ratio chi-square statistic: 128.214, two-tail p value: .0000 (based on 1 degree of freedom and 1222 complete observations).

INDEPENDENT VARIABLE	REGRESSION COEFFICIENT	STANDARD DEVIATION	CHI-SQUARE (DF = 1)	2-TAIL P VALUE	ODDS RATIO MULTIPLIER
intercept	-2.5921	.1550	279.6238	.0000	.0749
LOGUIRI	5.3948	.4897	121.3604	.0000	220.2619

GOODNESS OF STATISTICAL FIT OF LOGISTIC REGRESSION MODEL

Pearson chi-square fit statistic (based on 5 degrees of freedom): 2.950, p value: .7078.

Deviance chi-square fit statistic (based on 5 degrees of freedom): 3.060, p value: .6907.

The area under the complete ROC curve is estimated to be 0.7133.

****
Both the goodness-of-statistical-fit statistics and the chi-square value assigned to the LOGUIRI regression coefficient can be improved still further by partitioning the 278 undefined MITRATE values into separate subscales. As suggested in section 2.7, such partitioning is generally performed by means of

a routinely recorded patient attribute or index that appears to exert a large impact on the focal state or event. Primary tumor thickness, as divided by the AJCC into T1, T2, T3, and T4 categories, constitutes an appropriate partitioning index. The AJCC T-scale index is labeled AJCCTHIC. Based on its relative frequencies, when cross-tabulated with DSS5YR, an extended version of LOGUIRI is defined and labeled LOGUIRI1.

Another logistic regression analysis is performed, using LOGUIRI1 as the single independent variable and DSSDUMMY as the dependent variable. Both goodness-of-statistical-fit statistics suggest a slightly more reasonable fit of the logistic regression model with the extended impact-reflecting index numbers. The chi-square value assigned to the LOGUIRI1 regression coefficient is noticeably higher than the chi-square values assigned, respectively, to the MITRATE and LOGUIRI coefficients. Most interestingly, prediction of the focal event appears to be more accurate. The area under the complete ROC curve (AUC) increases from 0.7133 to 0.7524 (but beware the possibility of overfitting).
****

VALUE OF ATTRIBUTE AJCCTHIC	VALUE OF ATTRIBUTE DSS5YR		
	DSS>5YRS	MM DEATH=<5YRS	TOTAL
1	156	8	164
2	29	9	38
3	15	7	22
4	23	21	44
*	6	4	10
TOTAL	229	49	278

```
DEFINE LOGUIRI1:
18/234 IF MITRATE<2 ELSE
36/256 IF MITRATE>=2 AND MITRATE<4 ELSE
8/164 IF MITRATE=UNDEFN AND AJCCTHIC=1 ELSE
9/38 IF MITRATE=UNDEFN AND AJCCTHIC=2 ELSE
7/22 IF MITRATE=UNDEFN AND AJCCTHIC=3 ELSE
21/44 IF MITRATE=UNDEFN AND AJCCTHIC=4 ELSE
4/10 IF MITRATE=UNDEFN AND AJCCTHIC=UNDEFN ELSE
25/96 IF MITRATE=4 ELSE
51/145 IF MITRATE>=5 AND MITRATE<7 ELSE
59/127 IF MITRATE>=7 AND MITRATE<9 ELSE
43/86 IF MITRATE>=9
```

Numeric expression number 1 is just the attribute DSSDUMMY.
Numeric expression number 2 is just the attribute LOGUIRI1.

The effective working data set contains the 1222 PATIENTs constituting the DSSPROG WDS in the context DEC10.

After removing all undefined values from all expressions, the resulting number of PATIENTs for which each of the two expressions possesses a defined value is reduced to 1222. This constitutes the effective sample size.

RESULTS OF LOGISTIC REGRESSION ANALYSIS (LINEAR MODEL)

The dependent variable is a binary-coded numeric variable whose values are either 0 or 1. It is embodied in the first expression (parameter) of the LOGREG command, which is just the attribute DSSDUMMY.

The independent variable LOGUIRI1 is just the attribute LOGUIRI1.

Likelihood ratio chi-square statistic: 177.290, two-tail p value: .0000 (based on 1 degree of freedom and 1222 complete observations).

INDEPENDENT VARIABLE	REGRESSION COEFFICIENT	STANDARD DEVIATION	CHI-SQUARE (DF = 1)	2-TAIL P VALUE	ODDS RATIO MULTIPLIER
intercept	-2.7665	.1596	300.3680	.0000	.0629
LOGUIRI1	5.8037	.4657	155.3303	.0000	331.5100

GOODNESS OF STATISTICAL FIT OF LOGISTIC REGRESSION MODEL

Pearson chi-square fit statistic (based on 9 degrees of freedom): 5.277, p value: .8095.

Deviance chi-square fit statistic (based on 9 degrees of freedom): 5.477, p value: .7909.

The area under the complete ROC curve is estimated to be 0.7524.

****
The above analysis demonstrates how partitioning the subscale containing undefined values of some prognostic factor such as MITRATE into sub-subscales can improve predictive results. However, such improvements may come at a cost. Notice from the definition of LOGUIRI1 that only ten patient values fall into the sub-subscale containing undefined values of both MITRATE and AJCCTHIC. The related 40 percent estimate (4/10) of the incidence of MM death is, therefore, statistically unstable. Only when the sizes of all partitioned subscales and sub-subscales remain reasonably large is such partitioning advisable. Hence, LOGUIRI, rather than LOGUIRI1, will be used in the remainder of this appendix to avoid any possibility that the training data may have been so overfitted.

Now we analyze the same MITRATE prognostic factor via Cox regression. The dependent variable is the time elapsed (in years) between initial diagnosis and disease-specific death (i.e., due to metastatic melanoma). The same training sample of 1,222 melanoma patients used in the logistic regression is used in this Cox regression.

As outlined in section 2.7, the first step is to define six 0/1 dummy variables, one for each of the six defined partitions of the MITRATE scale. A multivariate Cox regression is then executed on these six dummy variables. An extra scale partition is reserved for the 278 missing observations.
****

The effective working data set contains the 1222 PATIENTs constituting the DSSPROG WDS in the context DEC10.

The effective sample size is 1222. This means that the number of PATIENTs contained within the effective WDS whose elapsed focal event or censored times are all strictly positive and all of whose independent variables possess defined values is 1222. The number of PATIENTs in the effective sample who experience the focal event is 409.

RESULTS OF COX REGRESSION ANALYSIS (PROPORTIONAL HAZARDS MODEL)

The dependent variable is either the time elapsed until the focal event occurs (focal event time), if the focal event does occur, or the time elapsed without the occurrence of the focal event (censored time), if the focal event has not yet occurred as of the latest observation. The dependent variable is embodied in the first two expressions (parameters) of the COXREG command shown below.

The first expression is DATEINT(DATEDIAG,DATEDIED) IF CAUSEOFD="METASTATIC MELANOMA" OR CAUSEOFD="MELANOSIS".
The second expression is DATEINT(DATEDIAG,DATELDSS).

The independent variable EXPRESSION3 is 1 IF MITRATE<2 ELSE 0.
The independent variable EXPRESSION4 is 1 IF MITRATE>=2 AND MITRATE<4 ELSE 0.
The independent variable EXPRESSION5 is 1 IF MITRATE=4 ELSE 0.
The independent variable EXPRESSION6 is 1 IF MITRATE>=5 AND MITRATE<7 ELSE 0.
The independent variable EXPRESSION7 is 1 IF MITRATE>=7 AND MITRATE<9 ELSE 0.
The independent variable EXPRESSION8 is 1 IF MITRATE>=9 ELSE 0.

Likelihood ratio chi-square statistic: 98.380, two-tail p value: .0000.
Score chi-square statistic: 106.564, two-tail p value: .0000.
Wald chi-square statistic: 96.529, two-tail p value: .0000.

All three chi-square statistics are based on 6 degrees of freedom and 1222 observations, encompassing 381 distinct focal event times.

INDEPENDENT VARIABLE	REGRESSION COEFFICIENT	STANDARD DEVIATION	CHI-SQUARE (DF = 1)	2-TAIL P VALUE	RELATIVE RISK
EXPRESSION3	-.6854	.1905	12.9466	.0003	.5039
EXPRESSION4	-.2145	.1641	1.7082	.1912	.8070
EXPRESSION5	.3013	.1968	2.3439	.1258	1.3516
EXPRESSION6	.4223	.1690	6.2459	.0124	1.5254
EXPRESSION7	.7889	.1641	23.1218	.0000	2.2009
EXPRESSION8	.8736	.1824	22.9490	.0000	2.3956

****
UIRI again stands for Univariate Impact-Reflecting Index, in this case designed as an independent variable for Cox regression analysis. Relative risks (hazard ratios) are first rescaled. Then, for each subscale in the partitioned MITRATE scale the UIRI is set equal to the natural logarithm of the rescaled relative risk assigned via Cox regression to the 0/1 dummy variable associated with all patients falling into that subscale. Dummy variables assign 1 to a patient for falling into a designated subscale or 0 for not falling into that subscale. This implements the procedure outlined in section 2.7 for Cox regression.
****

DEFINE COXUIRI:
0 IF MITRATE<2 ELSE
LOG(.8070/.5039) IF MITRATE>=2 AND MITRATE<4 ELSE
LOG(1.0000/.5039) IF MITRATE=UNDEFN ELSE
LOG(1.3516/.5039) IF MITRATE=4 ELSE
LOG(1.5254/.5039) IF MITRATE>=5 AND MITRATE<7 ELSE
LOG(2.2009/.5039) IF MITRATE>=7 AND MITRATE<9 ELSE
LOG(2.3956/.5039) IF MITRATE>=9

VALUE OF PARTITIONED MITRATE SCALE	VALUE OF ATTRIBUTE COXUIRI						
	.0000	.4709	.6854	.9867	1.1076	1.4742	1.5590	TOTAL
MITOTIC RATE 0 OR 1 per hpf	234	0	0	0	0	0	0	234
MITOTIC RATE 2 OR 3 per hpf	0	256	0	0	0	0	0	256
MITOTIC RATE UNDEFINED	0	0	278	0	0	0	0	278
MITOTIC RATE 4 per hpf	0	0	0	96	0	0	0	96
MITOTIC RATE 5 OR 6 per hpf	0	0	0	0	145	0	0	145
MITOTIC RATE 7 OR 8 per hpf	0	0	0	0	0	127	0	127
MITOTIC RATE AT LEAST 9 per hpf	0	0	0	0	0	0	86	86
TOTAL	234	256	278	96	145	127	86	1222

****

The same unidirectional pattern reflected in the values of LOGUIRI is likewise reflected in the values of COXUIRI. Lower values of COXUIRI are associated with DSS>5YRS, while higher values are associated with MM DEATH=<5YRS.

Separate Cox regression analyses are now performed, first on MITRATE (in its raw data form), and then on COXUIRI, the impact-reflecting index derived from MITRATE via the six-dummy-variable Cox regression just executed. In both analyses, the dependent variable is the time elapsed (in years) between initial diagnosis and disease-specific death (i.e., due to metastatic melanoma).

Once again, improved results are obtained in the second analysis from partitioning and "spacing" raw measurement values of the MITRATE scale to compute corresponding COXUIRI values.
****

Numeric expression number 1 is DATEINT(DATEDIAG,DATEDIED) IF CAUSEOFD= "METASTATIC MELANOMA" OR CAUSEOFD="MELANOSIS".
Numeric expression number 2 is DATEINT(DATEDIAG,DATELDSS).
Numeric expression number 3 is just the attribute MITRATE.

The effective working data set contains the 1222 PATIENTs constituting the DSSPROG WDS in the context DEC10.

The effective sample size is 944. This means that the number of PATIENTs contained within the effective WDS whose elapsed focal event or censored times are all strictly positive and all of whose independent variables possess defined values is 944. The number of PATIENTs in the effective sample who experience the focal event is 328.

RESULTS OF COX REGRESSION ANALYSIS (PROPORTIONAL HAZARDS MODEL)

The dependent variable is either the time elapsed until the focal event occurs (focal event time), if the focal event does occur, or the time elapsed without the occurrence of the focal event (censored time), if the focal event has not yet occurred as of the latest observation. The dependent variable is embodied in the first two expressions (parameters) of the COXREG command shown below.

The first expression is DATEINT(DATEDIAG,DATEDIED) IF CAUSEOFD="METASTATIC MELANOMA" OR CAUSEOFD="MELANOSIS".
The second expression is DATEINT(DATEDIAG,DATELDSS).

The independent variable MITRATE is just the attribute MITRATE.

Likelihood ratio chi-square statistic: 63.980, two-tail p value: .0000.

Score chi-square statistic: 82.990, two-tail p value: .0000.
Wald chi-square statistic: 81.050, two-tail p value: .0000.

All three chi-square statistics are based on 1 degree of freedom and 944
observations, encompassing 308 distinct focal event times.

INDEPENDENT VARIABLE	REGRESSION COEFFICIENT	STANDARD DEVIATION	CHI-SQUARE (DF = 1)	2-TAIL P VALUE	RELATIVE RISK
MITRATE	.1010	.0112	81.0503	.0000	1.1062

Numeric expression number 1 is DATEINT(DATEDIAG,DATEDIED) IF CAUSEOFD=
"METASTATIC MELANOMA" OR CAUSEOFD="MELANOSIS".
Numeric expression number 2 is DATEINT(DATEDIAG,DATELDSS).
Numeric expression number 3 is just the attribute COXUIRI.

The effective working data set contains the 1222 PATIENTs constituting the
DSSPROG WDS in the context DEC10.

The effective sample size is 1222. This means that the number of PATIENTS
contained within the effective WDS whose elapsed focal event or censored times
are all strictly positive and all of whose independent variables possess
defined values is 1222. The number of PATIENTs in the effective sample who
experience the focal event is 409.

RESULTS OF COX REGRESSION ANALYSIS (PROPORTIONAL HAZARDS MODEL)

The dependent variable is either the time elapsed until the focal event occurs
(focal event time), if the focal event does occur, or the time elapsed without
the occurrence of the focal event (censored time), if the focal event has not
yet occurred as of the latest observation. The dependent variable is embodied
in the first two expressions (parameters) of the COXREG command shown below.

The first expression is DATEINT(DATEDIAG,DATEDIED) IF CAUSEOFD="METASTATIC
MELANOMA" OR CAUSEOFD="MELANOSIS".
The second expression is DATEINT(DATEDIAG,DATELDSS).

The independent variable COXUIRI is just the attribute COXUIRI.

Likelihood ratio chi-square statistic: 98.380, two-tail p value: .0000.
Score chi-square statistic: 100.377, two-tail p value: .0000.
Wald chi-square statistic: 96.529, two-tail p value: .0000.

All three chi-square statistics are based on 1 degree of freedom and 1222
observations, encompassing 381 distinct focal event times.

INDEPENDENT VARIABLE	REGRESSION COEFFICIENT	STANDARD DEVIATION	CHI-SQUARE (DF = 1)	2-TAIL P VALUE	RELATIVE RISK
COXUIRI	1.0000	.1018	96.5289	.0000	2.7183

****
When a UIRI for Cox regression is calculated as described in section 2.7 and
illustrated above for MITRATE, its numeric values are natural logarithms of the
pairwise hazard ratios comparing each partitioned subscale of the prognostic
risk factor to its lowest-risk subscale. The ratio of the lowest-risk
subscale's hazard to itself is 1.0. Its logarithm is 0.0. Hence, for Cox
regression, the lowest-risk subscale is uniformly assigned a UIRI value of 0.0.
Values of all UIRIs for higher-risk subscales are larger positive numbers.

Normalization on a logarithmic hazard ratio scale has six pleasant consequences.

1. Regardless of the raw measurement scale of any prognostic factor, when converted to an equivalent Cox UIRI index, its UIRI scale will be directly comparable to the UIRI scales of all other converted factor indexes. By uniformly converting all factors to equivalent UIRIs, the relative risk characteristics of the respective subscales of any set of prognostic factors may be compared by visual inspection. Adjusting hazard ratios for disparate raw measurement scales is no longer necessary in judging which factors indicate higher or lower magnitudes of risk at various factor levels.

2. When an equivalent UIRI index is the single input to a univariate Cox regression whose end point (dependent variable) is the same as that used to construct the UIRI, the regression will always estimate a single regression coefficient of exactly one (see 1.0000 for the Cox regression of COXUIRI displayed toward the bottom of the previous page). This is a consequence of the construction procedure outlined in section 2.7. It can be used to verify that the construction procedure has been properly executed.

3. When two or more prognostic factors are first converted to equivalent Cox UIRIs, based on the same end point, and when the UIRIs are then submitted as independent variables to a multivariate Cox regression, also based on the same end point, the relative risks estimated by the analysis for each UIRI may also be compared directly and visually. By construction, all Cox UIRIs share the same scale. This permits comparing the relative impact potency (i.e., relative risks) of separate factors without having to adjust printed output statistics for disparate raw measurement scales.

4. The joint (combined) impact of any subset of prognostic factors may be estimated by constructing a weighted average Cox UIRI, using as weights the regression coefficients estimated by a multivariate Cox regression of the kind just described. The relative impacts of separate groups of prognostic factors may then be compared (e.g., traditional factors versus newly discovered factors).

5. When a joint (combined) UIRI is constructed as a weighted average UIRI of two or more prognostic factors and then used as the single input to a univariate Cox regression whose end point (dependent variable) is the same as that used to construct each component UIRI, the regression will always estimate a regression coefficient of exactly one. This, too, can be used to verify that the construction procedure has been properly executed to produce each component UIRI and the weighted average UIRI.

6. The fact that a univariate Cox regression of any single or joint (combined) UIRI uniformly generates an estimated regression coefficient of exactly one means that the constant of proportionality used to multiply a baseline hazard function to obtain an individual patient's hazard function in Cox (proportional hazards) regression may be interpreted as an exponentially weighted product of the component pairwise hazard ratios comparing each partitioned subscale of each prognostic risk factor to its lowest-risk subscale. For example, a patient whose value of a prognostic factor (all values in a set of factors in a joint index) falls within the lowest-risk subscale will possess a constant of proportionality exactly equal to one. This means that the shared baseline hazard function applies without modification to such a patient. Patients with one or more factor values falling in higher-risk subscales will possess a constant of proportionality greater than one, which serves both to elevate their individual hazard functions and to depress their individual survival functions compared to the respective baseline functions. Elevated or depressed and by how

        much for each component factor may now be calculated at a glance.

The COXREG command has been programmed to calculate and display values of the
estimated baseline survival function presumed to be shared by all patients in
the population from which the 1,222 melanoma patients were obtained. To compare
baseline survival rates with corresponding survival rates of a Kaplan-Meier
curve fitted to the same data, COXUIRI input values have been adjusted (i.e.,
converted to deviations from the training sample mean). This adjustment of
COXUIRI inputs affects only the level of estimated baseline functions. Nothing
else in the Cox regression analysis is altered.

Note the close agreement between Kaplan-Meier and baseline survival rates over
the entire range.

Following the parallel display columns is a report of an attempt to fit both an
exponential and a Weibull function, statistically, to the baseline hazard
function—also presumed to be shared by all patients in the population. The
baseline survival and hazard functions are mathematically related. Both the
exponential and the Weibull functions fit the data very well. The Weibull
function, with a slight decreasing trend in the baseline hazard rate over time,
fits slightly better (analogous R squared is approximately 96 percent).
****

COMPARISON OF KAPLAN-MEIER (PRODUCT LIMIT) AND BASELINE SURVIVAL RATES

ELAPSED TIME UNITS	NUMBER OF EVENTS	NUMBER AT RISK	KAPLAN-MEIER SURVIVAL RATE	BASELINE SURVIVAL RATE
0.0000	N/A	1222	1.0000	1.0000
.1670	1	1222	.9992	.9993
.2190	1	1221	.9984	.9986
.2272	1	1220	.9975	.9978
.2711	1	1219	.9967	.9971
.2847	1	1218	.9959	.9964
.3066	1	1217	.9951	.9956
.3258	1	1216	.9943	.9949
.4107	1	1215	.9935	.9942
.5093	1	1214	.9926	.9935
.5421	1	1213	.9918	.9927
.5531	1	1212	.9910	.9920
.5859	1	1211	.9902	.9913
.6133	1	1210	.9894	.9906
.6242	1	1209	.9885	.9898
.6379	1	1208	.9877	.9891
.6571	1	1207	.9869	.9884
.6790	1	1206	.9861	.9876
.6845	1	1205	.9853	.9869
.7201	1	1204	.9845	.9862
.7255	1	1203	.9836	.9855
.7474	1	1202	.9828	.9847
.7748	1	1201	.9820	.9840
.7913	1	1200	.9812	.9833
.7967	1	1199	.9804	.9825
.8049	1	1198	.9795	.9818
.8132	1	1197	.9787	.9811
.8159	1	1196	.9779	.9804
.8460	1	1195	.9771	.9796
.8597	1	1194	.9763	.9789

.8843	1	1193	.9755	.9782
.9008	1	1192	.9746	.9774
.9829	1	1191	.9738	.9767
.9856	1	1190	.9730	.9760
1.0075	1	1189	.9722	.9752
1.0185	2	1188	.9705	.9738
1.0240	1	1186	.9697	.9730
1.0267	2	1185	.9681	.9716
1.0404	1	1183	.9673	.9709
1.0815	1	1182	.9664	.9701
1.1089	1	1181	.9656	.9694
1.1143	1	1180	.9648	.9687
1.1171	1	1179	.9640	.9679
1.1308	2	1178	.9624	.9664
1.1444	1	1176	.9615	.9657
1.1581	1	1175	.9607	.9650
1.1773	1	1174	.9599	.9642
1.1965	2	1173	.9583	.9628
1.2047	2	1171	.9566	.9613
1.2102	1	1169	.9558	.9606
1.2129	2	1168	.9542	.9591
1.2156	1	1166	.9534	.9583
1.2184	1	1165	.9525	.9576
1.2238	1	1164	.9517	.9569
1.2375	1	1163	.9509	.9561
1.2622	2	1162	.9493	.9546
1.2649	1	1160	.9484	.9539
1.2813	1	1159	.9476	.9531
1.2950	1	1158	.9468	.9524
1.3005	2	1157	.9452	.9509
1.3142	1	1155	.9444	.9502
1.3306	1	1154	.9435	.9494
1.3416	1	1153	.9427	.9487
1.3471	1	1152	.9419	.9479
1.3799	1	1151	.9411	.9472
1.3909	1	1150	.9403	.9464
1.4264	1	1149	.9394	.9457
1.4429	2	1148	.9378	.9442
1.4511	1	1146	.9370	.9434
1.4675	1	1145	.9362	.9427
1.4703	1	1144	.9354	.9419
1.4922	1	1143	.9345	.9412
1.5305	2	1142	.9329	.9397
1.5360	1	1140	.9321	.9389
1.5442	1	1139	.9313	.9382
1.5469	2	1138	.9296	.9367
1.5633	1	1136	.9288	.9359
1.5688	1	1135	.9280	.9352
1.5852	1	1134	.9272	.9344
1.5880	1	1133	.9264	.9337
1.5962	1	1132	.9255	.9329
1.6126	2	1131	.9239	.9314
1.6510	1	1129	.9231	.9307
1.6619	1	1128	.9223	.9299
1.6674	1	1127	.9214	.9292
1.6920	1	1126	.9206	.9284
1.6948	1	1125	.9198	.9277
1.7002	1	1124	.9190	.9269
1.7085	2	1123	.9173	.9254

1.7194	1	1121	.9165	.9246
1.7221	1	1120	.9157	.9239
1.7276	1	1119	.9149	.9231
1.7440	1	1118	.9141	.9224
1.7988	1	1117	.9133	.9216
1.8015	1	1116	.9124	.9209
1.8234	1	1115	.9116	.9201
1.8344	1	1114	.9108	.9193
1.8371	2	1113	.9092	.9178
1.8508	1	1111	.9083	.9171
1.8590	1	1110	.9075	.9163
1.8782	1	1109	.9067	.9155
1.8837	1	1108	.9059	.9148
1.8864	1	1107	.9051	.9140
1.8892	1	1106	.9043	.9133
1.8946	1	1105	.9034	.9125
1.9111	1	1104	.9026	.9117
1.9193	1	1103	.9018	.9110
1.9247	2	1102	.9002	.9095
1.9384	1	1100	.8993	.9087
1.9439	1	1099	.8985	.9079
1.9686	1	1098	.8977	.9072
1.9822	2	1097	.8961	.9056
2.0041	1	1095	.8953	.9049
2.0178	1	1094	.8944	.9041
2.0288	1	1093	.8936	.9033
2.0452	1	1092	.8928	.9026
2.0562	1	1091	.8920	.9018
2.0808	2	1090	.8903	.9003
2.0835	1	1088	.8895	.8995
2.0918	1	1087	.8887	.8987
2.0945	1	1086	.8879	.8980
2.1000	1	1085	.8871	.8972
2.1082	1	1084	.8863	.8964
2.1164	1	1083	.8854	.8957
2.1821	1	1082	.8846	.8949
2.1903	1	1081	.8838	.8941
2.2204	1	1080	.8830	.8933
2.2341	1	1079	.8822	.8926
2.2478	1	1078	.8813	.8918
2.2615	1	1077	.8805	.8910
2.2779	2	1076	.8789	.8895
2.2916	2	1074	.8773	.8879
2.2998	1	1072	.8764	.8872
2.3628	1	1071	.8756	.8864
2.3683	1	1070	.8748	.8856
2.3738	1	1069	.8740	.8848
2.3765	1	1068	.8732	.8841
2.4230	1	1067	.8723	.8833
2.4313	1	1066	.8715	.8825
2.4614	1	1065	.8707	.8817
2.4669	1	1064	.8699	.8810
2.4723	1	1063	.8691	.8802
2.4970	1	1062	.8682	.8794
2.5216	1	1061	.8674	.8786
2.5599	1	1060	.8666	.8779
2.5682	1	1059	.8658	.8771
2.5846	1	1058	.8650	.8763
2.5901	1	1057	.8642	.8755

2.6065	1	1056	.8633	.8747
2.6421	2	1055	.8617	.8732
2.6722	1	1053	.8609	.8724
2.6859	1	1052	.8601	.8716
2.6968	1	1051	.8592	.8709
2.7023	1	1050	.8584	.8701
2.7324	1	1049	.8576	.8693
2.7352	1	1048	.8568	.8685
2.7625	1	1047	.8560	.8677
2.7735	1	1046	.8552	.8669
2.8009	1	1045	.8543	.8662
2.8036	1	1044	.8535	.8654
2.8146	1	1043	.8527	.8646
2.8283	1	1042	.8519	.8638
2.8392	1	1041	.8511	.8630
2.8611	1	1040	.8502	.8622
2.8967	1	1039	.8494	.8615
2.9104	1	1038	.8486	.8607
2.9213	1	1037	.8478	.8599
2.9241	1	1036	.8470	.8591
2.9296	1	1035	.8462	.8583
2.9350	1	1034	.8453	.8575
2.9460	1	1033	.8445	.8568
2.9706	1	1032	.8437	.8560
2.9734	2	1031	.8421	.8544
2.9898	2	1029	.8404	.8528
2.9980	2	1027	.8388	.8513
3.0226	1	1025	.8380	.8505
3.0391	1	1024	.8372	.8497
3.0418	1	1023	.8363	.8489
3.0665	1	1022	.8355	.8481
3.0692	1	1021	.8347	.8473
3.1020	1	1020	.8339	.8465
3.1185	1	1019	.8331	.8457
3.1349	1	1018	.8322	.8450
3.1376	1	1017	.8314	.8442
3.1924	2	1016	.8298	.8426
3.2417	1	1014	.8290	.8418
3.2526	1	1013	.8282	.8410
3.2581	1	1012	.8273	.8402
3.3320	1	1011	.8265	.8394
3.3402	1	1010	.8257	.8386
3.3485	1	1009	.8249	.8378
3.3539	1	1008	.8241	.8371
3.3594	1	1007	.8232	.8363
3.3813	1	1006	.8224	.8355
3.3841	1	1005	.8216	.8347
3.3868	1	1004	.8208	.8339
3.4114	1	1003	.8200	.8331
3.4142	1	1002	.8191	.8323
3.4196	1	1001	.8183	.8315
3.4470	1	1000	.8175	.8307
3.4580	1	999	.8167	.8299
3.4635	1	998	.8159	.8291
3.4662	1	997	.8151	.8284
3.4908	1	996	.8142	.8276
3.5018	1	995	.8134	.8268
3.5894	1	994	.8126	.8260
3.6195	1	993	.8118	.8252

3.6442	1	992	.8110	.8244
3.6551	1	991	.8101	.8236
3.6825	1	990	.8093	.8228
3.6962	1	989	.8085	.8220
3.6989	1	988	.8077	.8212
3.7071	1	987	.8069	.8204
3.7236	1	986	.8061	.8196
3.7290	1	985	.8052	.8188
3.8084	1	984	.8044	.8180
3.8166	1	983	.8036	.8172
3.8249	1	982	.8028	.8164
3.8385	1	981	.8020	.8156
3.8522	1	980	.8011	.8148
3.8550	1	979	.8003	.8141
3.8714	1	978	.7995	.8133
3.8769	1	977	.7987	.8125
3.9070	1	976	.7979	.8117
3.9152	1	975	.7971	.8109
3.9289	1	974	.7962	.8101
3.9837	1	973	.7954	.8093
4.0302	1	972	.7946	.8085
4.0412	1	971	.7938	.8077
4.0548	1	970	.7930	.8069
4.0822	1	969	.7921	.8061
4.0850	1	968	.7913	.8053
4.1507	1	967	.7905	.8045
4.1808	1	966	.7897	.8037
4.2164	1	965	.7889	.8029
4.2547	1	964	.7881	.8021
4.2602	1	963	.7872	.8013
4.3013	1	962	.7864	.8005
4.4053	1	961	.7856	.7997
4.4573	1	960	.7848	.7989
4.4655	1	959	.7840	.7981
4.4683	1	958	.7831	.7972
4.5066	1	957	.7823	.7964
4.5093	1	956	.7815	.7956
4.5778	1	955	.7807	.7948
4.5997	1	954	.7799	.7940
4.6161	1	953	.7791	.7932
4.6271	1	952	.7782	.7924
4.6435	1	951	.7774	.7916
4.6462	1	950	.7766	.7908
4.6709	1	949	.7758	.7900
4.6818	1	948	.7750	.7892
4.7202	1	947	.7741	.7884
4.7421	1	946	.7733	.7876
4.7996	1	945	.7725	.7868
4.8105	1	944	.7717	.7860
4.8844	1	943	.7709	.7851
4.9939	1	942	.7700	.7843
5.0104	1	941	.7692	.7835
5.0241	1	939	.7684	.7827
5.0268	1	938	.7676	.7819
5.0350	1	937	.7668	.7811
5.2376	1	910	.7659	.7803
5.2568	2	909	.7642	.7786
5.2595	2	906	.7626	.7769
5.2951	1	900	.7617	.7761

5.3033	1	899	.7609	.7752
5.3608	1	890	.7600	.7744
5.4566	1	876	.7591	.7735
5.4703	1	874	.7583	.7727
5.5169	1	869	.7574	.7718
5.5963	1	863	.7565	.7709
5.6374	1	860	.7556	.7701
5.6401	1	858	.7548	.7692
5.6812	1	852	.7539	.7683
5.7031	1	850	.7530	.7674
5.7469	1	846	.7521	.7666
5.7907	1	840	.7512	.7657
5.8181	1	837	.7503	.7648
5.8345	1	832	.7494	.7639
5.9166	2	826	.7476	.7621
5.9413	1	821	.7467	.7612
5.9632	1	814	.7458	.7603
6.0371	1	806	.7448	.7594
6.0426	1	805	.7439	.7585
6.0480	1	803	.7430	.7575
6.0727	1	801	.7421	.7566
6.0918	1	800	.7411	.7557
6.0973	1	799	.7402	.7548
6.1220	1	796	.7393	.7539
6.2315	1	783	.7383	.7529
6.2835	1	777	.7374	.7520
6.2999	1	775	.7364	.7510
6.3027	1	774	.7355	.7501
6.3574	1	762	.7345	.7491
6.3684	1	760	.7335	.7482
6.3930	1	757	.7326	.7472
6.4450	1	751	.7316	.7462
6.4724	1	749	.7306	.7453
6.5053	1	741	.7296	.7443
6.5135	1	739	.7286	.7433
6.6257	1	724	.7276	.7423
6.6778	1	716	.7266	.7413
6.7024	1	709	.7256	.7403
6.7654	1	704	.7246	.7392
6.8010	1	699	.7235	.7382
6.8256	1	694	.7225	.7372
6.8283	1	693	.7214	.7361
6.9488	1	675	.7204	.7351
6.9762	1	673	.7193	.7340
7.0282	1	663	.7182	.7330
7.0665	1	659	.7171	.7319
7.1186	1	654	.7160	.7308
7.2527	1	636	.7149	.7297
7.3376	1	630	.7138	.7286
7.4937	1	601	.7126	.7274
7.4991	1	599	.7114	.7262
7.5375	1	593	.7102	.7250
7.6744	1	576	.7090	.7238
7.7674	1	570	.7077	.7226
7.8112	1	563	.7065	.7213
7.8989	1	551	.7052	.7200
7.9126	1	548	.7039	.7187
7.9153	1	547	.7026	.7174
8.1699	1	519	.7013	.7161

8.3451	1	499	.6999	.7147
8.4519	1	489	.6984	.7132
8.5012	1	485	.6970	.7118
8.5724	1	477	.6955	.7104
8.6737	1	468	.6940	.7089
8.6764	1	467	.6925	.7074
8.7011	1	466	.6911	.7059
8.7257	1	463	.6896	.7045
8.7394	1	461	.6881	.7030
8.7695	1	456	.6866	.7015
8.7723	1	455	.6851	.7000
8.9009	1	440	.6835	.6984
9.0269	1	430	.6819	.6968
9.0762	1	427	.6803	.6952
9.1720	1	419	.6787	.6936
9.2623	1	412	.6770	.6919
9.3719	1	401	.6754	.6902
9.4704	1	391	.6736	.6885
9.4923	2	388	.6702	.6850
9.5033	1	384	.6684	.6833
9.5745	1	376	.6666	.6815
9.6101	1	372	.6648	.6797
9.7333	1	360	.6630	.6779
9.7908	1	355	.6611	.6760
9.8099	1	350	.6592	.6741
9.8181	1	349	.6573	.6722
9.9441	1	345	.6554	.6703
9.9742	1	342	.6535	.6684
10.1987	1	326	.6515	.6664
10.2097	1	324	.6495	.6644
10.2425	1	323	.6475	.6624
10.3958	1	306	.6454	.6603
10.5492	1	294	.6432	.6581
10.6340	1	287	.6409	.6558
10.6368	1	285	.6387	.6536
10.8010	1	272	.6363	.6513
11.0858	1	258	.6339	.6488
11.1132	1	257	.6314	.6463
11.2802	1	246	.6288	.6438
11.3076	1	241	.6262	.6411
11.3760	1	237	.6236	.6385
11.6826	1	219	.6207	.6356
11.7155	1	218	.6179	.6328
11.8907	1	207	.6149	.6298
12.2083	1	187	.6116	.6265
12.7532	1	166	.6079	.6228
12.9613	1	159	.6041	.6190
13.6895	1	132	.5995	.6144
13.7251	1	130	.5949	.6099
13.7279	1	129	.5903	.6053
13.8730	1	123	.5855	.6006
14.4890	1	98	.5795	.5949
15.3131	1	76	.5719	.5874
15.5650	1	71	.5639	.5794
15.7895	1	65	.5552	.5705
16.7505	1	49	.5439	.5587
18.1742	1	34	.5279	.5399

TOTAL   409

If the population of elapsed time intervals until an event occurs is assumed to follow an exponential distribution, implying a constant hazard rate throughout every observation subwindow, the maximum likelihood estimate of the ordinary hazard rate is .042208, with a standard error of .002087.

The assumption of an exponential distribution with a constant hazard rate produces a *VERY GOOD* fit with the observed data. The analogue of an unadjusted coefficient of determination (R squared) would be .9259.

If the population of elapsed time intervals until an event occurs is assumed to follow a Weibull distribution, which permits either an increasing or a decreasing hazard rate over all observation subwindows, the maximum likelihood estimate of the ordinary intensity parameter (analogous to the constant ordinary hazard rate parameter characterizing an exponential distribution) is .038635, with a standard error of .002745. In addition, there appears to be a *DECREASING* trend in the hazard rate over time. The maximum likelihood estimate of the ordinary trend parameter is .913588, with a standard error of .040617.

The assumption of a Weibull distribution with a *DECREASING* hazard rate produces a better fit with the data—at least in this complete observation window (two-tail p value: .0334). The improved value of the analogue of an unadjusted coefficient of determination (R squared) is .9567, indicating an *EXTREMELY GOOD* fit.

If the population of elapsed time intervals until an event occurs is assumed to follow an exponential distribution, implying a constant hazard rate throughout every observation subwindow, the maximum likelihood estimate of the *BASELINE* hazard rate is .040057, with a standard error of .001981.

The assumption of an exponential distribution with a constant hazard rate produces a *VERY GOOD* fit with the observed data. The analogue of an unadjusted coefficient of determination (R squared) would be .9420.

If the population of elapsed time intervals until an event occurs is assumed to follow a Weibull distribution, which permits either an increasing or a decreasing hazard rate over all observation subwindows, the maximum likelihood estimate of the *BASELINE* intensity parameter (analogous to the constant *BASELINE* hazard rate parameter characterizing an exponential distribution) is .037626, with a standard error of .002669. In addition, there appears to be a *DECREASING* trend in the hazard rate over time. The maximum likelihood estimate of the *BASELINE* trend parameter is .942345, with a standard error of .041072.

The assumption of a Weibull distribution with a *DECREASING* hazard rate produces a better fit with the data—at least in this complete observation window (two-tail p value: .1604). The improved value of the analogue of an unadjusted coefficient of determination (R squared) is .9595, indicating an *EXTREMELY GOOD* fit.

* *
Since Cox regression was performed on adjusted values of COXUIRI as its single independent variable and because the estimated value of the regression coefficient was 1.0, define HAZPROP for each patient as the exponentiated value of that patient's adjusted COXUIRI value. HAZPROP is each patient's estimated constant of proportionality embodying the proportional hazards assumption underlying Cox regression.
* *

DEFINE HAZPROP: EXP{1*[COXUIRI-MEAN(COXUIRI)]}

SUMMARY STATISTICS	ATTRIBUTE HAZPROP
n DEFINED	1222
MINIMUM	.4836
MEDIAN	.9598
MAXIMUM	2.2992
MEAN	1.1302
STD. DEV.	.5701

VALUE OF ATTRIBUTE HAZPROP	ABSOLUTE FREQUENCIES (COUNTS)	RELATIVE FREQUENCIES (PROPORTIONS)	CUMULATIVE RELATIVE FREQUENCIES
.4836	234	.1915	.1915
.7745	256	.2095	.4010
.9598	278	.2275	.6285
1.2972	96	.0786	.7070
1.4640	145	.1187	.8257
2.1123	127	.1039	.9296
2.2992	86	.0704	1.0000
TOTAL	1222	1.0000	

****
Define LOGPROB as the individually tailored probability of MM DEATH=<5YRS
estimated by the logistic regression of DSSDUMMY on LOGUIRI.

Define COXPROB as the complement of the individually tailored fitted survival
probability function obtained from Cox regression and evaluated for each
patient at an elapsed time of five years.

Since LOGPROB and COXPROB are conceptually equivalent, although calculated
under somewhat different assumptions implying different mathematical models,
each patient's LOGPROB and COXPROB probabilities should be approximately equal.
As shown in the table below, they are reasonably close, except that LOGPROB
values rise more quickly than the corresponding COXPROB values when MITRATE
exceeds 5 per hbf. Furthermore, they are extremely highly linearly correlated
(r = .98) and perfectly rank-order correlated (r = 1.00).
****

DEFINE LOGPROB: EXP(-2.5921+5.3948*LOGUIRI)/[1+EXP(-2.5921+5.3948*LOGUIRI)]
DEFINE COXPROB: 1-EXP{-HAZPROP*[.037626*5]^.942345}

VALUE OF ATTRIBUTE LOGPROB	VALUE OF ATTRIBUTE COXPROB							
	.0953	.1482	.1803	.2356	.2616	.3544	.3789	TOTAL
.1018	234	0	0	0	0	0	0	234
.1378	0	256	0	0	0	0	0	256
.1623	0	0	278	0	0	0	0	278
.2338	0	0	0	96	0	0	0	96
.3330	0	0	0	0	145	0	0	145
.4785	0	0	0	0	0	127	0	127
.5263	0	0	0	0	0	0	86	86
TOTAL	234	256	278	96	145	127	86	1222

The value of the Pearson product-moment (linear) correlation coefficient is .9800.

This observed correlation coefficient displays an *EXTREMELY SIGNIFICANT DIRECTIONAL DEPARTURE* from what would be expected if the sample of paired expression values had been drawn from a bivariate normally distributed population with a true correlation of zero.

Significance test results: one-tail p-value (directional alternate hypothesis) is .0000, and two-tail p-value (nondirectional alternate hypothesis) is .0000.

The value of the Spearman rank-order correlation coefficient is 1.0000.

It is more convenient to test statistical significance by means of the equivalent Kendall Tau rank-order correlation coefficient calculated from the same pair of expressions. This is done below.

The value of the Kendall Tau rank-order correlation coefficient is 1.0000.

This observed correlation coefficient displays an *EXTREMELY SIGNIFICANT DIRECTIONAL DEPARTURE* from what would be expected if the sample of paired expression values had been drawn from any population with a true rank-order correlation of zero.

Significance test results: one-tail p-value (directional alternate hypothesis) is .0000, and two-tail p-value (nondirectional alternate hypothesis) is .0000.

****
We are finally ready to assess predictive accuracy.

Because LOGPROB and COXPROB are perfectly rank-order correlated, there can be no difference in the AUC achieved by these two predictors under a ROC analysis. Neither can there be any difference in the maximum possible number of correct predictions for the same reason.
****

Standard ASCII string expression number 1 is just the attribute DSS5YR. Numeric expression number 2 is just the attribute LOGPROB.

The effective working data set contains the 1222 PATIENTs constituting the DSSPROG WDS in the context DEC10.

The first two expressions (parameters) in the command specification are completely defined on 1222 PATIENTs. This constitutes the effective sample size of the overall analysis.

2 distinct values of the first expression in the command specification and 7 distinct values of the second expression are defined for the effective sample.

Analysis will focus on the state or event identified as MM DEATH=<5YRS. The alternative state or event is identified as DSS>5YRS. Sample 2, containing 281 PATIENTs, is in the focal MM DEATH=<5YRS category, while sample 1, containing 941 PATIENTs, is in the alternative DSS>5YRS category.

The optimal cut point is .2338. It is optimal in the sense that it maximizes the average of the sensitivity and the specificity proportions achieved by any cut point. When their value of LOGPROB is at least .2338, PATIENTs are predicted as MM DEATH=<5YRS. When their value of LOGPROB is less than .2338, PATIENTs are predicted as DSS>5YRS. Using this binary cut point, the average of the sensitivity and the specificity proportions achieves a maximum value of .6701.

The area under the complete ROC curve is estimated to be .7133.

The maximum possible number of correct predictions is 941 out of 1222. This is equivalent to 77.0 percent correct.

Standard ASCII string expression number 1 is just the attribute DSS5YR. Numeric expression number 2 is just the attribute COXPROB.

The effective working data set contains the 1222 PATIENTs constituting the DSSPROG WDS in the context DEC10.

The first two expressions (parameters) in the command specification are completely defined on 1222 PATIENTs. This constitutes the effective sample size of the overall analysis.

2 distinct values of the first expression in the command specification and 7 distinct values of the second expression are defined for the effective sample.

Analysis will focus on the state or event identified as MM DEATH=<5YRS. The alternative state or event is identified as DSS>5YRS. Sample 2, containing 281 PATIENTs, is in the focal MM DEATH=<5YRS category, while sample 1, containing 941 PATIENTs, is in the alternative DSS>5YRS category.

The optimal cut point is .2356. It is optimal in the sense that it maximizes the average of the sensitivity and the specificity proportions achieved by any cut point. When their value of COXPROB is at least .2356, PATIENTs are predicted as MM DEATH=<5YRS. When their value of COXPROB is less than .2356, PATIENTs are predicted as DSS>5YRS. Using this binary cut point, the average of the sensitivity and the specificity proportions achieves a maximum value of .6701.

The area under the complete ROC curve is estimated to be .7133.

The maximum possible number of correct predictions is 941 out of 1222. This is equivalent to 77.0 percent correct.

****
A matched-pairs T test comparing the absolute individual prediction errors generated by using LOGPROB versus COXPROB as the predictor shows virtually no difference. The small difference between them is statistically insignificant.

This is encouraging. Even though corresponding LOGPROB and COXPROB probabilities were only approximately equal, the impact of these differences on absolute individual prediction errors tended to balance out. On the average, there was virtually no difference.
****

Numeric expression number 1 is ABS(DSSDUMMY-LOGPROB)-ABS(DSSDUMMY-COXPROB).

The effective working data set contains the 1222 PATIENTs constituting the DSSPROG WDS in the context DEC10.

SUMMARY STATISTICS	EXPRESSION NUMBER 1
n DEFINED	1222
MINIMUM	-.1474
MEDIAN	-.0065
MAXIMUM	.1474
MEAN	.0002
STD. DEV.	.0620

The computed mean of the sample of observations shown in the above table of summary statistics displays a *SLIGHT, BUT INSIGNIFICANT DIRECTIONAL DEPARTURE* from what would be expected if that sample had been drawn from a population whose true mean value were zero. The observed departure is in the POSITIVE direction.

A one-sample T test was performed on the above data.

The value of the T statistic is .11 with 1221 degrees of freedom.

Significance test results: one-tail p-value (directional alternate hypothesis) is .4573, and two-tail p-value (nondirectional alternate hypothesis) is .9145.

****

Appendix B

Attributes of the 1,222 Patients Included within the Melanoma Training Sample

In all the following tables, "*" signifies undefined (missing) observations.

```
SUMMARY              ATTRIBUTE
STATISTICS           AGE

n DEFINED                 1222
MINIMUM                      2
MEDIAN                      51
MAXIMUM                     89
MEAN                   51.5286
STD. DEV.              15.5846
```

VALUE OF DEFINING EXPRESSION	VALUE OF ATTRIBUTE AJCCAGE									TOTAL
	1	2	3	4	5	6	7	8	*	
10 =< AGE < 20 years old	16	0	0	0	0	0	0	0	0	16
20 =< AGE < 30 years old	0	81	0	0	0	0	0	0	0	81
30 =< AGE < 40 years old	0	0	187	0	0	0	0	0	0	187
40 =< AGE < 50 years old	0	0	0	282	0	0	0	0	0	282
50 =< AGE < 60 years old	0	0	0	0	252	0	0	0	0	252
60 =< AGE < 70 years old	0	0	0	0	0	228	0	0	0	228
70 =< AGE < 80 years old	0	0	0	0	0	0	138	0	0	138
AGE >= 80 years old	0	0	0	0	0	0	0	36	0	36
*	0	0	0	0	0	0	0	0	2	2
TOTAL	16	81	187	282	252	228	138	36	2	1222

Note: The two patients with undefined AJCCAGE were less than ten years old.

VALUE OF ATTRIBUTE AJCCAGE	ABSOLUTE FREQUENCIES (COUNTS)	RELATIVE FREQUENCIES (PROPORTIONS)	CUMULATIVE RELATIVE FREQUENCIES
1	16	.0131	.0131
2	81	.0663	.0794
3	187	.1530	.2324
4	282	.2308	.4632
5	252	.2062	.6694
6	228	.1866	.8560
7	138	.1129	.9689
8	36	.0295	.9984
*	2	.0016	1.0000
TOTAL	1222	1.0000	

VALUE OF ATTRIBUTE SEX	ABSOLUTE FREQUENCIES (COUNTS)	RELATIVE FREQUENCIES (PROPORTIONS)	CUMULATIVE RELATIVE FREQUENCIES
FEMALE	479	.3920	.3920
MALE	743	.6080	1.0000
TOTAL	1222	1.0000	

VALUE OF DEFINING EXPRESSION	VALUE OF ATTRIBUTE AJCCSEX		
	0	1	TOTAL
FEMALE	479	0	479
MALE	0	743	743
TOTAL	479	743	1222

VALUE OF ATTRIBUTE TUMPLACE	ABSOLUTE FREQUENCIES (COUNTS)	RELATIVE FREQUENCIES (PROPORTIONS)	CUMULATIVE RELATIVE FREQUENCIES
HEADNECK	268	.2193	.2193
HIGHEXT	187	.1530	.3723
LOWEXT	274	.2242	.5966
TRUNK	487	.3985	.9951
*	6	.0049	1.0000
TOTAL	1222	1.0000	

Note: TUMPLACE designates the anatomical location of the patient's primary tumor. There were six missing observations.

VALUE OF ATTRIBUTE TUMPLACE	VALUE OF ATTRIBUTE AJCCSITE			
	0	1	*	TOTAL
HEADNECK	0	268	0	268
HIGHEXT	187	0	0	187
LOWEXT	274	0	0	274
TRUNK	0	487	0	487
*	0	0	6	6
TOTAL	461	755	6	1222

SUMMARY STATISTICS	ATTRIBUTE TUMTHICK
n DEFINED	1212
MINIMUM	.0500
MEDIAN	1.7000
MAXIMUM	35.0000
MEAN	2.9261
STD. DEV.	3.3091

VALUE OF DEFINING EXPRESSION	VALUE OF ATTRIBUTE AJCCTHIC					
	1	2	3	4	*	TOTAL
T1: 0 < TUMTHICK =< 1 mm.	392	0	0	0	0	392
T2: 1 < TUMTHICK =< 2 mm.	0	290	0	0	0	290
T3: 2 < TUMTHICK =< 4 mm.	0	0	229	0	0	229
T4: TUMTHICK > 4 mm.	0	0	0	301	0	301
*	0	0	0	0	10	10
TOTAL	392	290	229	301	10	1222

Note: There were ten missing observations.

VALUE OF ATTRIBUTE TUMTHICK	ABSOLUTE FREQUENCIES (COUNTS)	RELATIVE FREQUENCIES (PROPORTIONS)	CUMULATIVE RELATIVE FREQUENCIES
.05	2	.0016	.0016
.15	3	.0025	.0041
.20	5	.0041	.0082
.25	3	.0025	.0106
.29	1	.0008	.0115
.30	12	.0098	.0213
.34	1	.0008	.0221
.35	6	.0049	.0270
.40	17	.0139	.0409
.42	1	.0008	.0417
.45	6	.0049	.0466
.50	29	.0237	.0704
.53	1	.0008	.0712
.55	4	.0033	.0745
.60	25	.0205	.0949
.62	1	.0008	.0957
.65	7	.0057	.1015
.68	1	.0008	.1023
.70	38	.0311	.1334
.72	1	.0008	.1342
.75	17	.0139	.1481
.76	2	.0016	.1498
.78	1	.0008	.1506
.80	41	.0336	.1841
.82	1	.0008	.1849
.84	1	.0008	.1858
.85	11	.0090	.1948
.88	2	.0016	.1964
.89	1	.0008	.1972
.90	39	.0319	.2291
.92	2	.0016	.2308
.93	1	.0008	.2316
.95	20	.0164	.2480
.96	1	.0008	.2488
.98	2	.0016	.2504
1.00	86	.0704	.3208
1.03	1	.0008	.3216
1.05	2	.0016	.3232
1.10	27	.0221	.3453
1.15	4	.0033	.3486
1.17	1	.0008	.3494
1.20	38	.0311	.3805
1.25	5	.0041	.3846
1.28	1	.0008	.3854
1.30	32	.0262	.4116
1.35	4	.0033	.4149
1.40	27	.0221	.4370
1.45	5	.0041	.4411
1.50	24	.0196	.4607
1.55	2	.0016	.4624
1.60	27	.0221	.4845
1.65	6	.0049	.4894
1.67	1	.0008	.4902
1.70	19	.0155	.5057
1.75	2	.0016	.5074

1.80	21	.0172	.5245
1.85	2	.0016	.5262
1.90	7	.0057	.5319
1.95	1	.0008	.5327
2.00	31	.0254	.5581
2.10	14	.0115	.5696
2.20	24	.0196	.5892
2.24	1	.0008	.5900
2.25	2	.0016	.5917
2.30	11	.0090	.6007
2.35	2	.0016	.6023
2.37	1	.0008	.6031
2.40	15	.0123	.6154
2.50	22	.0180	.6334
2.60	8	.0065	.6399
2.64	1	.0008	.6408
2.65	1	.0008	.6416
2.70	10	.0082	.6498
2.75	4	.0033	.6530
2.80	7	.0057	.6588
2.90	4	.0033	.6620
3.00	22	.0180	.6800
3.10	5	.0041	.6841
3.20	11	.0090	.6931
3.30	4	.0033	.6964
3.40	6	.0049	.7013
3.50	16	.0131	.7144
3.55	2	.0016	.7160
3.60	5	.0041	.7201
3.70	4	.0033	.7234
3.80	5	.0041	.7275
4.00	22	.0180	.7455
4.10	8	.0065	.7520
4.20	17	.0139	.7660
4.25	1	.0008	.7668
4.30	11	.0090	.7758
4.40	3	.0025	.7782
4.50	17	.0139	.7921
4.60	6	.0049	.7971
4.70	1	.0008	.7979
4.80	10	.0082	.8061
4.90	1	.0008	.8069
5.00	30	.0245	.8314
5.10	2	.0016	.8331
5.20	3	.0025	.8355
5.30	1	.0008	.8363
5.40	2	.0016	.8380
5.50	19	.0155	.8535
5.60	3	.0025	.8560
5.70	1	.0008	.8568
5.80	4	.0033	.8601
6.00	25	.0205	.8805
6.20	1	.0008	.8813
6.40	1	.0008	.8822
6.50	19	.0155	.8977
6.60	3	.0025	.9002
6.75	1	.0008	.9010
7.00	21	.0172	.9182
7.10	2	.0016	.9198

7.20	5	.0041	.9239
7.30	1	.0008	.9247
7.50	8	.0065	.9313
7.70	1	.0008	.9321
7.80	1	.0008	.9329
7.90	2	.0016	.9345
8.00	12	.0098	.9444
9.00	8	.0065	.9509
9.50	5	.0041	.9550
9.80	1	.0008	.9558
10.00	7	.0057	.9615
10.30	1	.0008	.9624
10.50	1	.0008	.9632
11.00	6	.0049	.9681
12.00	7	.0057	.9738
13.00	3	.0025	.9763
14.00	3	.0025	.9787
14.40	1	.0008	.9795
14.50	1	.0008	.9804
15.00	3	.0025	.9828
16.00	1	.0008	.9836
19.00	1	.0008	.9845
20.00	5	.0041	.9885
25.00	1	.0008	.9894
30.00	1	.0008	.9902
35.00	2	.0016	.9918
*	10	.0082	1.0000
TOTAL	1222	1.0000	

VALUE OF ATTRIBUTE CLARKLEV	ABSOLUTE FREQUENCIES (COUNTS)	RELATIVE FREQUENCIES (PROPORTIONS)	CUMULATIVE RELATIVE FREQUENCIES
I	4	.0033	.0033
II	93	.0761	.0794
III	390	.3191	.3985
IV	455	.3723	.7709
V	131	.1072	.8781
*	149	.1219	1.0000
TOTAL	1222	1.0000	

Note: There were 149 missing observations.

VALUE OF DEFINING EXPRESSION	1	2	3	4	5	*	TOTAL
CLARK LEVEL I	4	0	0	0	0	0	4
CLARK LEVEL II	0	93	0	0	0	0	93
CLARK LEVEL III	0	0	390	0	0	0	390
CLARK LEVEL IV	0	0	0	455	0	0	455
CLARK LEVEL V	0	0	0	0	131	0	131
*	0	0	0	0	0	149	149
TOTAL	4	93	390	455	131	149	1222

VALUE OF ATTRIBUTE AJCCLARK

```
SUMMARY              ATTRIBUTE
STATISTICS            MITRATE

n DEFINED              944
MINIMUM                  0
MEDIAN                   3
MAXIMUM                 22
MEAN                 4.2044
STD. DEV.            3.6542
```

VALUE OF ATTRIBUTE MITRATE	ABSOLUTE FREQUENCIES (COUNTS)	RELATIVE FREQUENCIES (PROPORTIONS)	CUMULATIVE RELATIVE FREQUENCIES
0	74	.0606	.0606
1	160	.1309	.1915
2	145	.1187	.3101
3	111	.0908	.4010
4	96	.0786	.4795
5	119	.0974	.5769
6	26	.0213	.5982
7	56	.0458	.6440
8	71	.0581	.7021
9	11	.0090	.7111
10	21	.0172	.7283
11	1	.0008	.7291
12	26	.0213	.7504
13	2	.0016	.7520
14	2	.0016	.7537
15	5	.0041	.7578
16	3	.0025	.7602
18	12	.0098	.7700
22	3	.0025	.7725
*	278	.2275	1.0000
TOTAL	1222	1.0000	

Note: MITRATE (mitotic rate) is a count of mitoses observed in a high-powered
      microscopic field (hpf) interpreted as one square millimeter at UCSF.
      There were 278 missing observations.

VALUE OF DEFINING EXPRESSION	VALUE OF ATTRIBUTE AJCCMITR			
	0	1	*	TOTAL
0 per hpf	74	0	0	74
1 per hpf	0	160	0	160
2 per hpf	0	145	0	145
3 per hpf	0	111	0	111
4 per hpf	0	96	0	96
5 per hpf	0	119	0	119
6 per hpf	0	26	0	26
7 per hpf	0	56	0	56
8 per hpf	0	71	0	71
9 per hpf	0	11	0	11
10 per hpf	0	21	0	21
11 per hpf	0	1	0	1
12 per hpf	0	26	0	26
13 per hpf	0	2	0	2

```
14 per hpf          0      2      0            2
15 per hpf          0      5      0            5
16 per hpf          0      3      0            3
18 per hpf          0     12      0           12
22 per hpf          0      3      0            3
*                   0      0    278          278

   TOTAL           74    870    278         1222
```

Note: In 2009 the AJCC recommended that partitioning the mitotic rate scale in
      the above manner was appropriate for prognostic purposes, especially for
      distinguishing between 1a and 1b patients in their staging criteria.

VALUE OF ATTRIBUTE ULCERATN	ABSOLUTE FREQUENCIES (COUNTS)	RELATIVE FREQUENCIES (PROPORTIONS)	CUMULATIVE RELATIVE FREQUENCIES
NO	711	.5818	.5818
YES	324	.2651	.8470
*	187	.1530	1.0000
TOTAL	1222	1.0000	

Note: ULCERATN signifies presence or absence of ulceration of the primary
      tumor. There were 187 missing observations.

TABLE OF JOINT ABSOLUTE FREQUENCIES (COUNTS)

VALUE OF ATTRIBUTE ULCERATN	VALUE OF ATTRIBUTE AJCCULC			
	0	1	*	TOTAL
NO	711	0	0	711
YES	0	324	0	324
*	0	0	187	187
TOTAL	711	324	187	1222

VALUE OF ATTRIBUTE FIRSTAGE	ABSOLUTE FREQUENCIES (COUNTS)	RELATIVE FREQUENCIES (PROPORTIONS)	CUMULATIVE RELATIVE FREQUENCIES
1a	78	.0638	.0638
1b	322	.2635	.3273
2a	105	.0859	.4133
2b	94	.0769	.4902
2c	63	.0516	.5417
3a	51	.0417	.5835
3b	138	.1129	.6964
3c	161	.1318	.8282
4	7	.0057	.8339
*	203	.1661	1.0000
TOTAL	1222	1.0000	

Note: FIRSTAGE is AJCC Stage at the time of initial patient diagnosis. There
      were 203 missing observations.

VALUE OF ATTRIBUTE TUMTYPE	ABSOLUTE FREQUENCIES (COUNTS)	RELATIVE FREQUENCIES (PROPORTIONS)	CUMULATIVE RELATIVE FREQUENCIES
ACRAL	43	.0352	.0352
DESMOPLASTIC	48	.0393	.0745
LENTIGO MALIGNANT MELANOMA	32	.0262	.1007
MALIGNANT MELANOMA IN NEVUS	1	.0008	.1015
MELANOMA IN PIGMENTED NEVUS	1	.0008	.1023
OTHER/NOT OTHERWISE CLASSIFIED	113	.0925	.1948
MUCOSAL	1	.0008	.1956
NODULAR	251	.2054	.4010
SPINDLE CELL	2	.0016	.4026
SUPERFICIAL SPREADING	464	.3797	.7823
UVEAL	1	.0008	.7831
*	265	.2169	1.0000
TOTAL	1222	1.0000	

Note: TUMTYPE designates the histologic type of the patient's primary tumor. There were 265 missing observations.

Appendix C

Relative Prognostic Weights in Differentiating the Incidence of MM DEATH=<5YRS
Generated by Least-Squares Weighting Rescaled Univariate Impact Probabilities

PROGNOSTIC RISK FACTOR	LOW-RISK PATIENTS INCIDENCE = 5.37% SAMPLE SIZE = 503	MEDIUM-RISK PATIENTS INCIDENCE = 24.59% SAMPLE SIZE = 423	HIGH-RISK PATIENTS INCIDENCE = 50.68% SAMPLE SIZE = 296
AGE (years)	W/D	.3942	W/D
SEX (male/female)	.0745	.0000	.0000
AJCC PRIMARY SITE	.0000	.0000	.0000
THICKNESS (mm.)	.2850	.1030	.1863
MITOTIC RATE (/hpf)	.6405	.5028	.6919
ULCERATION (yes/no)	W/D	.0000	.1218
FACTOR GROUP TOTAL	1.0000	1.0000	1.0000
TUMOR TYPE	.0000	.0000	.0427
CLARK LEVEL (1 to 5)	.7179	.0000	.0000
ANGIOGENESIS (0 to 3)	.2821	.0052	.4467
TIL LEVEL (0 to 3)	W/D	.0000	.0000
MICROSATELLITES (yes/no)	I/D	.0000	.0683
VASC. INVOLV. (yes/no)	I/D	.6558	.0000
REGRESSION (0 to 2)	W/D	.0000	W/D
INITIAL AJCC STAGE	.0000	.3390	.0000
POSITIVE NODE COUNT	I/D	.0000	.4423
FACTOR GROUP TOTAL	1.0000	1.0000	1.0000
WNT2 (RWS 0-3 scale)	W/D	.0000	W/D
ARPC2 (RWS 0-3 scale)	W/D	.0000	.0000
OPN (RWS 0-3 scale)	.0000	.0000	W/D
RGS1 (RWS 0-3 scale)	.0000	.7612	.2158
FN1 (RWS 0-3 scale)	.6774	.2094	.6032
NCOA3 (RWS 0-3 scale)	.0000	.0000	W/D
P65 (RWS 0-3 scale)	.0000	W/D	W/D
PHIP (RWS 0-3 scale)	.3226	.0294	.1810
POU5 (RWS 0-3 scale)	.0000	.0000	.0000
FACTOR GROUP TOTAL	1.0000	1.0000	1.0000

Optimally Differentiating Binary Cut Points for Univariate Impact Probabilities

Differentiating Factors Used to Define Separate Risk Levels

THICKNESS (mm.)	1.30/1.35	2.70/2.75	4.20/4.25
POSITIVE NODE COUNT	I/D	0/1	1/2
INITIAL AJCC STAGE	1a/1b	3a/3b	2c/3c

Nondefinitional Differentiating Factors with Increasing Cut Points

MITOTIC RATE (/hpf)	3/4	4/5	4/5
PHIP (RWS 0-3 scale)	1/2	2/3	2/3

Nondefinitional Differentiating Factor with Stable Cut Point

CLARK LEVEL	III/IV	III/IV	III/IV

Explanatory Notes:

1. I/D means that the prognostic risk factor possessed insufficient data to support a differentiating analysis at that risk level (e.g., no low-risk patients possessed either any MICROSATELLITES or any positive lymph nodes).
2. W/D means that the prognostic factor pointed statistically insignificantly in the wrong direction for patients at that risk level. Thus, ULCERATION was uniformly involved via AJCC staging in stratifying patients according to their underlying risk level and, therefore, was a potent overall prognostic factor; but it pointed insignificantly in the wrong direction for low-risk patients and insignificantly in the right direction for medium-risk patients and significantly in the right direction for high-risk patients.
3. The nine gene-based molecular markers in the third factor group are still regarded as relatively novel prognostic factors. Nevertheless, enough prior research has been performed so that they, like the other fifteen factors, may be regarded as possessing a known "risky" versus "nonrisky" direction. Prior research has shown that relative overexpression of all nine molecular markers points in the "risky" direction, while their relative underexpression points in the "nonrisky" direction (designated W/D).
4. A weight of .0000 means that the prognostic factor did point in the right direction for patients at that risk level, but either it provided too weak a signal or it was too tightly correlated with other, more strongly prognostic factors within the same factor group to receive a positive weight indicating its independent, relative within-group, differentiating prognostic potency.
5. An optimally differentiating (within that factor group) binary cut point X/Y means between the X and Y values on the scale of that risk factor.
6. The AJCC reports that the optimally differentiating cut point for DSS within their sample of T1 patients used to distinguish between the T1A and T1B categories was 0/1 on the MITOTIC RATE scale. Most of their T1 patients were T1A. Most of our T1 patients were T1B. All fifty-four of our T1A patients whose MITOTIC RATE was recorded possessed a zero MITOTIC RATE, while all but three of our 168 T1B patients whose MITOTIC RATE was recorded possessed a positive MITOTIC RATE. The same 0/1 cut point, but only for our T1 patients, supports the observation that MITOTIC RATE is a prognostic risk factor whose optimally differentiating cut points regularly increase with increasing patient risk level, in contrast to the stable cut point for CLARK LEVEL.
7. When the three factor groups were merged, differentiating prognostic potency weights for low-risk patients were as follows:

```
MITOTIC RATE            .5380
CLARK LEVEL             .4620

LOW-RISK TOTAL         1.0000
```

8. Imagine that a low-risk patient is freshly diagnosed. Assume that low-risk patient is fairly typical in the sense that all six AJCC traditional factors, plus TUMOR TYPE, CLARK LEVEL, and INITIAL AJCC STAGE, have been properly assessed at the time of diagnosis. That leaves the remaining six of the second (histological) factor group and all nine of the third (molecular) factor group nonassessed. The differentiating prognostic potency weights for these fifteen remaining, nonassessed risk factors would be as follows:

```
ANGIOGENESIS            .4806
FN1                     .5077
PHIP                    .0117

NONASSESSED TOTAL      1.0000
```

9. When the three factor groups were merged, differentiating prognostic potency
   weights for medium-risk patients were as follows:

   ```
   AGE                     .2848
   MITOTIC RATE            .3834
   VASC. INVOLV.           .2563
   RGS1                    .0755

   MEDIUM-RISK TOTAL    1.0000
   ```

10. Imagine that a medium-risk patient is freshly diagnosed. Assume that
    medium-risk patient is fairly typical in the sense that all six AJCC
    traditional factors, plus TUMOR TYPE, CLARK LEVEL, and INITIAL AJCC STAGE,
    have been properly assessed at the time of diagnosis. That leaves the
    remaining six of the second (histological) factor group and all nine of the
    third (molecular) factor group nonassessed. The differentiating prognostic
    potency weights for these fifteen remaining, nonassessed risk factors would
    be as follows:

    ```
    VASC. INVOLV.           .5584
    RGS1                    .4416

    NONASSESSED TOTAL    1.0000
    ```

11. When the three factor groups were merged, differentiating prognostic
    potency weights for high-risk patients were as follows:

    ```
    MITOTIC RATE            .3383
    ANGIOGENESIS            .2930
    POSITIVE NODE COUNT     .3687

    HIGH-RISK TOTAL    1.0000
    ```

12. Imagine that a high-risk patient is freshly diagnosed. Assume that
    high-risk patient is fairly typical in the sense that all six AJCC
    traditional factors, plus TUMOR TYPE, CLARK LEVEL, and INITIAL AJCC STAGE,
    have been properly assessed at the time of diagnosis. That leaves the
    remaining six of the second (histological) factor group and all nine of the
    third (molecular) factor group nonassessed. The differentiating prognostic
    potency weights for these fifteen remaining, nonassessed risk factors would
    be as follows:

    ```
    ANGIOGENESIS            .4613
    MICROSATELLITES         .0829
    POSITIVE NODE COUNT     .4558

    NONASSESSED TOTAL    1.0000
    ```

Appendix D

Attributes of the 1,225 Patients in the Breast Cancer Training Sample

In all the following tables, "*" signifies undefined (missing) observations.

SUMMARY STATISTICS	ATTRIBUTE AGEDIAG
n DEFINED	1225
MINIMUM	24
MEDIAN	57
MAXIMUM	97
MEAN	57.6253
STD. DEV.	12.4150

Note: AGEDIAG means age at diagnosis in years as of last birthday.

VALUE OF DEFINING EXPRESSION	VALUE OF ATTRIBUTE CONVAGE							TOTAL
	2	3	4	5	6	7	8	
20 =< AGEDIAG < 30 years old	5	0	0	0	0	0	0	5
30 =< AGEDIAG < 40 years old	0	82	0	0	0	0	0	82
40 =< AGEDIAG < 50 years old	0	0	271	0	0	0	0	271
50 =< AGEDIAG < 60 years old	0	0	0	322	0	0	0	322
60 =< AGEDIAG < 70 years old	0	0	0	0	315	0	0	315
70 =< AGEDIAG < 80 years old	0	0	0	0	0	189	0	189
AGEDIAG >= 80 years old	0	0	0	0	0	0	41	41
TOTAL	5	82	271	322	315	189	41	1225

Note: To be as comparable as possible with the way the AJCC treated the age of melanoma patients at diagnosis, the conventional age index (CONVAGE) was defined for breast cancer patients as shown above. There were no missing observations.

VALUE OF ATTRIBUTE CONVAGE	ABSOLUTE FREQUENCIES (COUNTS)	RELATIVE FREQUENCIES (PROPORTIONS)	CUMULATIVE RELATIVE FREQUENCIES
2	5	.0041	.0041
3	82	.0669	.0710
4	271	.2212	.2922
5	322	.2629	.5551
6	315	.2571	.8122
7	189	.1543	.9665
8	41	.0335	1.0000
TOTAL	1225	1.0000	

VALUE OF ATTRIBUTE CONVSEX	ABSOLUTE FREQUENCIES (COUNTS)	RELATIVE FREQUENCIES (PROPORTIONS)	CUMULATIVE RELATIVE FREQUENCIES
0	1225	1.0000	1.0000
TOTAL	1225	1.0000	

Note: All 1,225 patients were female, so the conventional sex index (CONVSEX) was defined as shown above to remain comparable with the AJCC definition of AJCCSEX. There were no missing observations.

VALUE OF ATTRIBUTE TUMPLACE	ABSOLUTE FREQUENCIES (COUNTS)	RELATIVE FREQUENCIES (PROPORTIONS)	CUMULATIVE RELATIVE FREQUENCIES
CENTRAL	158	.1290	.1290
DIFFUSE	42	.0343	.1633
LATERAL	619	.5053	.6686
MEDIAL	214	.1747	.8433
*	192	.1567	1.0000
TOTAL	1225	1.0000	

Note: TUMPLACE designates the anatomical location in the breast of the patient's primary tumor.

VALUE OF ATTRIBUTE TUMPLACE	VALUE OF ATTRIBUTE CONVSITE			
	0	1	*	TOTAL
CENTRAL	0	158	0	158
DIFFUSE	0	42	0	42
LATERAL	619	0	0	619
MEDIAL	214	0	0	214
*	0	0	192	192
TOTAL	833	200	192	1225

Note: CONVSITE is the conventional site index defined to remain comparable with the AJCC definition of AJCCSITE. There were 192 missing observations.

VALUE OF ATTRIBUTE TUMORSIZ	ABSOLUTE FREQUENCIES (COUNTS)	RELATIVE FREQUENCIES (PROPORTIONS)	CUMULATIVE RELATIVE FREQUENCIES
5	9	.0073	.0073
6	2	.0016	.0090
8	1	.0008	.0098
9	1	.0008	.0106
10	73	.0596	.0702
12	5	.0041	.0743
13	3	.0024	.0767
15	61	.0498	.1265
16	1	.0008	.1273
18	3	.0024	.1298
19	14	.0114	.1412
20	124	.1012	.2424

21	5	.0041	.2465
25	37	.0302	.2767
29	2	.0016	.2784
30	153	.1249	.4033
31	2	.0016	.4049
35	20	.0163	.4212
39	1	.0008	.4220
40	58	.0473	.4694
45	7	.0057	.4751
50	49	.0400	.5151
51	4	.0033	.5184
60	37	.0302	.5486
61	7	.0057	.5543
65	1	.0008	.5551
70	20	.0163	.5714
71	2	.0016	.5731
75	2	.0016	.5747
80	12	.0098	.5845
81	1	.0008	.5853
100	5	.0041	.5894
101	1	.0008	.5902
*	502	.4098	1.0000
TOTAL	1225	1.0000	

Note: TUMORSIZ is the size of the patient's primary tumor in millimeters along its largest dimension. There were 502 missing observations.

DEFINE CONVSIZE: &
1 IF TUMORSIZ<20 ELSE &
2 IF TUMORSIZ=20 ELSE &
3 IF TUMORSIZ>=21 AND TUMORSIZ<40 ELSE &
4 IF TUMORSIZ>=40

The CONVSIZE index was defined as shown above to remain comparable with the AJCC tumor thickness index (AJCCTHIC). Optimal cut points for CONVSIZE were determined by applying the SPSA algorithm to the raw TUMORSIZ data. Again, this resulted in 502 missing observations.

VALUE OF ATTRIBUTE TUMORSIZ	VALUE OF ATTRIBUTE CONVSIZE					
	1	2	3	4	*	TOTAL
5	9	0	0	0	0	9
6	2	0	0	0	0	2
8	1	0	0	0	0	1
9	1	0	0	0	0	1
10	73	0	0	0	0	73
12	5	0	0	0	0	5
13	3	0	0	0	0	3
15	61	0	0	0	0	61
16	1	0	0	0	0	1
18	3	0	0	0	0	3
19	14	0	0	0	0	14
20	0	124	0	0	0	124
21	0	0	5	0	0	5
25	0	0	37	0	0	37
29	0	0	2	0	0	2
30	0	0	153	0	0	153

31	0	0	2	0	0	2
35	0	0	20	0	0	20
39	0	0	1	0	0	1
40	0	0	0	58	0	58
45	0	0	0	7	0	7
50	0	0	0	49	0	49
51	0	0	0	4	0	4
60	0	0	0	37	0	37
61	0	0	0	7	0	7
65	0	0	0	1	0	1
70	0	0	0	20	0	20
71	0	0	0	2	0	2
75	0	0	0	2	0	2
80	0	0	0	12	0	12
81	0	0	0	1	0	1
100	0	0	0	5	0	5
101	0	0	0	1	0	1
*	0	0	0	0	502	502
TOTAL	173	124	220	206	502	1225

Raw data for MITCOUNT (mitotic rate) in the sample of 1,225 breast cancer patients are shown below. There were no missing observations.

VALUE OF DEFINING EXPRESSION	VALUE OF ATTRIBUTE MITCOUNT			
	1	2	3	TOTAL
1: rare (0 or 1 mitoses per hpf)	474	0	0	474
2: 2 or 3 mitoses per hpf	0	476	0	476
3: more than 3 mitoses per hpf	0	0	275	275
TOTAL	474	476	275	1225

Note: MITCOUNT (mitotic rate) is a count of mitoses observed in a high-powered microscopic field (hpf).

The SPSA algorithm was applied to these data to obtain an optimal binary cut point. Using this cut point, the conventional index, CONVMITC, was defined to remain comparable with the AJCC index, AJCCMITR. Again, there were no missing observations.

VALUE OF ATTRIBUTE MITCOUNT	VALUE OF ATTRIBUTE CONVMITC		
	0	1	TOTAL
1	474	0	474
2	0	476	476
3	0	275	275
TOTAL	474	751	1225

VALUE OF DEFINING EXPRESSION	VALUE OF ATTRIBUTE ULCERATN			
	0	1	*	TOTAL
0 means no ulceration	1179	0	0	1179
1 means ulceration	0	42	0	42
*	0	0	4	4
TOTAL	1179	42	4	1225

Note: ULCERATN signifies presence or absence of ulceration of the primary tumor.

The CONVULC index was defined as identical to the raw ULCERATN attribute. There were four missing observations.

Initial staging data were unavailable for the 1,225 breast cancer patients.

T-scale, N-scale, and M-scale summary statistics are shown below.

SUMMARY STATISTICS	ATTRIBUTE T	ATTRIBUTE N	ATTRIBUTE M
n DEFINED	1209	1174	1225
MINIMUM	0	0	0
MEDIAN	2	0	0
MAXIMUM	4	3	1
MEAN	2.0794	.5784	.0759
STD. DEV.	.9566	.6383	.2649

VALUE OF ATTRIBUTE T	ABSOLUTE FREQUENCIES (COUNTS)	RELATIVE FREQUENCIES (PROPORTIONS)	CUMULATIVE RELATIVE FREQUENCIES
0	5	.0041	.0041
1	344	.2808	.2849
2	560	.4571	.7420
3	150	.1224	.8645
4	150	.1224	.9869
*	16	.0131	1.0000
TOTAL	1225	1.0000	

Note: There were sixteen missing observations.

VALUE OF ATTRIBUTE N	ABSOLUTE FREQUENCIES (COUNTS)	RELATIVE FREQUENCIES (PROPORTIONS)	CUMULATIVE RELATIVE FREQUENCIES
0	589	.4808	.4808
1	493	.4024	.8833
2	90	.0735	.9567
3	2	.0016	.9584
*	51	.0416	1.0000
TOTAL	1225	1.0000	

Note: There were fifty-one missing observations.

VALUE OF ATTRIBUTE M	ABSOLUTE FREQUENCIES (COUNTS)	RELATIVE FREQUENCIES (PROPORTIONS)	CUMULATIVE RELATIVE FREQUENCIES
0	1132	.9241	.9241
1	93	.0759	1.0000
TOTAL	1225	1.0000	

VALUE OF DEFINING EXPRESSION	VALUE OF ATTRIBUTE GRADE			
	1	2	3	TOTAL
1 means low grade	272	0	0	272
2 means medium grade	0	541	0	541
3 means high grade	0	0	412	412
TOTAL	272	541	412	1225

Note: GRADE means grade of primary tumor. There were no missing observations.

VALUE OF DEFINING EXPRESSION	VALUE OF ATTRIBUTE BILATERL			
	0	1	*	TOTAL
0 means no bilateral breast cancer	1137	0	0	1137
1 means bilateral breast cancer	0	85	0	85
*	0	0	3	3
TOTAL	1137	85	3	1225

Note: There were three missing observations.

VALUE OF ATTRIBUTE TUMTYPE	ABSOLUTE FREQUENCIES (COUNTS)	RELATIVE FREQUENCIES (PROPORTIONS)	CUMULATIVE RELATIVE FREQUENCIES
DUCTAL	1027	.8384	.8384
LOBULAR	198	.1616	1.0000
TOTAL	1225	1.0000	

Note: TUMTYPE means type of primary tumor.

VALUE OF ATTRIBUTE SURGTYPE	ABSOLUTE FREQUENCIES (COUNTS)	RELATIVE FREQUENCIES (PROPORTIONS)	CUMULATIVE RELATIVE FREQUENCIES
ABLATION	105	.0857	.0857
ABLATION + CLND (MODIFIED RADICAL)	292	.2384	.3241
BIOPSY	10	.0082	.3322
LUMPECTOMY + CLND	19	.0155	.3478
RADICAL MASTECTOMY (HALSTEDT)	795	.6490	.9967
*	4	.0033	1.0000
TOTAL	1225	1.0000	

Note: SURGTYPE means type of surgery. CLND means complete lymph node
      dissection. There were four missing observations.

VALUE OF DEFINING EXPRESSION	VALUE OF ATTRIBUTE RADIOTX			
	0	1	*	TOTAL
0 means no radiation therapy	304	0	0	304
1 means radiation therapy	0	919	0	919
*	0	0	2	2
TOTAL	304	919	2	1225

Note: RADIOTX indicates whether or not the patient was given any locoregional radiation therapy. There were two missing observations.

VALUE OF ATTRIBUTE ADJUVNTX	ABSOLUTE FREQUENCIES (COUNTS)	RELATIVE FREQUENCIES (PROPORTIONS)	CUMULATIVE RELATIVE FREQUENCIES
OVARIAN ABLATION	59	.0482	.0482
CMF	14	.0114	.0596
NO ADJUVANT THERAPY	807	.6588	.7184
OTHER ADJUVANT THERAPY	9	.0073	.7257
TAMOXIFEN	31	.0253	.7510
*	305	.2490	1.0000
TOTAL	1225	1.0000	

Note: ADJUVNTX means type of adjuvant therapy, if any, given to the patient. CMF means cyclophosphamide, methotrexate, and 5-fluoronracil. There were 305 missing observations.

Appendix E

Relative Prognostic Weights in Differentiating the Incidence of MBC DEATH=<5YRS
Generated by Least-Squares Weighting Rescaled Univariate Impact Probabilities

PROGNOSTIC RISK FACTOR	LOW-RISK PATIENTS INCIDENCE = 11.41% SAMPLE SIZE = 552	MEDIUM-RISK PATIENTS INCIDENCE = 39.79% SAMPLE SIZE = 387	HIGH-RISK PATIENTS INCIDENCE = 80.07% SAMPLE SIZE = 286
AGE (years)	.2338	W/D	.0000
SEX (all female)	I/D	I/D	I/D
BREAST TUMOR SITE	.0000	.0000	.3254
TUMOR SIZE (mm.)	.0941	.3153	.0000
MIT. COUNT (1-3 scale)	.6721	.6847	.6746
ULCERATION (yes/no)	I/D	I/D	.0000
FACTOR GROUP TOTAL	1.0000	1.0000	1.0000
LOBULAR/DUCTAL TUMOR	.0000	.0000	.0000
TUMOR GRADE (1-3 scale)	.5253	.6340	.7221
NECROSIS (0-3 scale)	.3457	.3660	.0000
TUB. FORM. (1-3 scale)	.0000	.0000	.0000
PLEOMORPH. (1-3 scale)	.0000	.0000	.0000
INFLAMMATION (yes/no)	I/D	I/D	.0000
ER (fmol./mg. index)	.0000	.0000	.0000
PR (fmol./mg. index)	.0000	.0000	I/D
BILATERALITY (yes/no)	W/D	W/D	W/D
T0 -> T4 T SCALE	.0735	.0000	W/D
N0 -> N3 N SCALE	.0555	.0000	.0000
M0 -> M1 M SCALE	I/D	I/D	.2779
FACTOR GROUP TOTAL	1.0000	1.0000	1.0000
RADIATION (yes/no)	1.0000	.3238	.5554
TYPE OF ADJ. THERAPY	I/D	.6762	.4446
FACTOR GROUP TOTAL	1.0000	1.0000	1.0000

Optimally Differentiating Binary Cut Points for Univariate Impact Probabilities

Differentiating Factors Used to Define Separate Risk Levels

T SCALE	1/2	1/2	W/D
N SCALE	0/1	0/1	1/2
M SCALE	I/D	I/D	0/1

Nondefinitional Differentiating Factors with Increasing Cut Points

AGE	69/70	W/D	73/74
TUMOR SIZE	25/30	35/40	60/61
GRADE	1/2	2/3	2/3

Nondefinitional Differentiating Factors with Stable Cut Points

MITOTIC COUNT	1/2	1/2	1/2
NECROSIS	0/1	0/1	0/1
TUB. FORM.	2/3	2/3	2/3
PLEOMORPH.	2/3	2/3	2/3

Explanatory Notes:

1. I/D means that the prognostic risk factor possessed insufficient data to support a differentiating analysis, at least at that indicated risk level (e.g., all patients at all risk levels were female, neither low-risk nor medium-risk patients had ulcerated primary tumors, while they all were M0 at the time of their original diagnosis and presented without inflammation).
2. W/D means that the prognostic factor pointed statistically insignificantly in the wrong direction for patients at that risk level. AGE at diagnosis pointed statistically insignificantly in the wrong direction for medium-risk patients, as did BILATERALITY for all patients at all risk levels.
3. A weight of .0000 means that the prognostic factor did point in the right direction for patients at that risk level, but either it provided too weak a signal or it was too tightly correlated with other, more strongly prognostic factors within the same factor group to receive a positive weight indicating its independent, relative within-group, differentiating prognostic potency. DUCTAL versus LOBULAR type of tumor was such a prognostic factor at all three risk levels, as were TUBULE FORMATION, PLEOMORPHISM, and ER.
4. An optimally differentiating (within that factor group) binary cut point X/Y means between the X and Y values on the scale of that risk factor.
5. When the three factor groups were merged, differentiating prognostic potency weights for low-risk patients were as follows:

AGE	.2201
TUMOR SIZE	.0444
MITOTIC COUNT	.6075
NECROSIS	.1280
LOW-RISK TOTAL	1.0000

6. Imagine that a low-risk patient is freshly diagnosed. Assume that low-risk patient is fairly typical in the sense that all of the five traditional factors, plus TUMOR TYPE and values on the T, N, and M scales, have been properly assessed at the time of diagnosis. That leaves the remaining eight factors in the second factor group nonassessed prior to therapy. The differentiating prognostic potency weights for these eight remaining, nonassessed, nontherapeutic risk factors, plus MITOTIC COUNT, would be as follows:

MITOTIC COUNT	.6530
TUMOR GRADE	.0581
NECROSIS	.2889
NONASSESSED TOTAL	1.0000

7. MITOTIC COUNT is an essential component of TUMOR GRADE. Consequently, the above weights, excluding a separate assessment of MITOTIC COUNT, would be altered as follows:

TUMOR GRADE	.5797
NECROSIS	.4203
NONASSESSED TOTAL	1.0000

8. When the three factor groups were merged, differentiating prognostic potency weights for medium-risk patients were as follows:

```
TUMOR SIZE              .1203
MITOTIC COUNT           .1452
TUMOR GRADE             .4908
NECROSIS                .2437

MEDIUM-RISK TOTAL    1.0000
```

9. Imagine that a medium-risk patient is freshly diagnosed. Assume that medium-risk patient is fairly typical in the sense that all of the five traditional factors, plus TUMOR TYPE and values on the T, N, and M scales, have been properly assessed at the time of diagnosis. That leaves the eight remaining factors in the second factor group nonassessed prior to therapy. The differentiating prognostic potency weights for these eight remaining, nonassessed, nontherapeutic risk factors, plus MITOTIC COUNT, would be as follows:

```
MITOTIC COUNT           .1684
TUMOR GRADE             .5172
NECROSIS                .3144

NONASSESSED TOTAL    1.0000
```

10. MITOTIC COUNT is an essential component of TUMOR GRADE. Consequently, the above weights, excluding a separate assessment of MITOTIC COUNT, would be altered as follows:

```
TUMOR GRADE             .6340
NECROSIS                .3660

NONASSESSED TOTAL    1.0000
```

11. When the three factor groups were merged, differentiating prognostic potency weights for high-risk patients were as follows:

```
TUMOR SITE              .1373
MITOTIC COUNT           .1525
TUMOR GRADE             .5779
M SCALE                 .1323

HIGH-RISK TOTAL      1.0000
```

12. Imagine that a high-risk patient is freshly diagnosed. Assume that high-risk patient is fairly typical in the sense that all of the five traditional factors, plus TUMOR TYPE and values on the T, N, and M scales, have been properly assessed at the time of diagnosis. That leaves the remaining eight factors in the second factor group nonassessed prior to therapy. The differentiating prognostic potency weights for these eight remaining, nonassessed, nontherapeutic risk factors, plus MITOTIC COUNT, would be as follows:

```
MITOTIC COUNT        .3171
TUMOR GRADE          .5956
TUBULE FORMATION     .0873

NONASSESSED TOTAL    1.0000
```

13. MITOTIC COUNT is an essential component of TUMOR GRADE. Consequently, the above weights, excluding a separate assessment of MITOTIC COUNT, would be altered as follows:

```
TUMOR GRADE          .8313
NECROSIS             .1190
TUBULE FORMATION     .0497

NONASSESSED TOTAL    1.0000
```

Appendix F

Two Limited-Scope, Split-Sample Reliability Analyses Designed
to Replicate and Validate PCM's Superior Predictive Accuracy

Our 1,222 melanoma patients were randomly partitioned into a training subsample
of 800 and a validation subsample of 422. Similarly, our 1,225 breast cancer
patients were randomly partitioned into a training subsample of 800 and a
validation subsample of 425. The procedures described in section 3 and section
4 were then applied, respectively, to the two training subsamples of 800
patients each.

To eliminate the risk of overfitting, the scope of these analyses was limited
to include only the six AJCC traditional prognostic factors in melanoma and the
corresponding five conventional factors used to predict breast cancer.

The goal of the split-sample analyses was to reproduce in the two 800-patient
training subsamples PCM's superior predictive accuracy, as reported in sections
3 and 4 for the two complete samples, and then to use prediction algorithms
generated from the training subsamples to reproduce PCM's superior predictive
accuracy in each validation subsample.

In only one detail did execution of these split-sample analyses differ from the
procedures reported in sections 3 and 4 for the two complete samples. Missing
data were handled differently in generating the prediction algorithms for the
practice-centered base cases, based solely on dummy-variable logistic
regression analyses of AJCC stage at diagnosis.

The two split-sample analyses were designed to illustrate our recommended
large-scale replication project for PCM. The three "artificial" risk subgroups
established for each complete sample in sections 3 and 4 would not exist in the
large-scale replication. There would be enough data to stratify each complete
sample, its training subsample, and its validation subsample into at least as
many distinct risk subgroups as there emerged distinguishable (i.e.,
statistically significantly different, in a prognostic sense) stages of disease
progression identified by the AJCC. Neither of these split-sample analyses
could anticipate how many such strata would eventually emerge. Consequently, an
additional "stratum" was created to contain all patients for each
practice-centered base case training subsample whose AJCC stage at diagnosis
could not be determined.

Three prediction algorithms were then generated from the 800-patient melanoma
training subsample in the following manner.

1. The first algorithm produced individually tailored probabilities of
   experiencing MM DEATH within five years of initial diagnosis. These
   probabilities constituted the factor-centered base case. They emerged
   from a standard (unstratified) logistic regression analysis of the six
   AJCC traditional prognostic factors, wherein missing observations of
   each factor were replaced by the mean value of that factor in the
   800-patient training subsample.

   Corresponding probabilities for the complete sample of 1,222 melanoma
   patients were labeled N5YRDPR in section 3. The ROC curve associated
   with N5YRDPR probabilities was the lowest one in Figure 7.

   Factor-centered base case probabilities in the training subsample
   yielded an estimated AUC of 0.7546. AUC was estimated as 0.7624 for the
   factor-centered base case in the complete 1,222-patient sample.

2. The second algorithm produced similar probabilities based solely on a dummy-variable logistic regression analysis of AJCC stage at initial diagnosis. These probabilities constituted the practice-centered base case, wherein missing observations of AJCC stage at diagnosis were replaced as just described for split-sample analysis.

   Corresponding probabilities for the complete sample of 1,222 melanoma patients were labeled F5YRDPR in section 3. The ROC curve associated with F5YRDPR probabilities was the second-lowest one in Figure 7.

   Practice-centered base case probabilities in the training subsample yielded an estimated AUC of 0.7832. AUC was estimated as 0.7867 for the practice-centered base case in the complete 1,222-patient sample.

3. The third algorithm produced similar probabilities based on a composite logistic regression analysis stratified by AJCC stage at diagnosis (PCM). Missing observations of each factor were replaced by PCM as described in sections 2.5, 2.6, and 2.7.

   Corresponding probabilities for the complete sample of 1,222 melanoma patients were labeled S5YRDPR in section 3. The ROC curve associated with S5YRDPR probabilities was the third-lowest one (second from the top) in Figure 7.

   PCM-generated probabilities in the training subsample yielded an estimated AUC of 0.8199. AUC was estimated as 0.8208 for PCM in the complete 1,222-patient sample.

4. In the training subsample, the PCM-based predictions improved AUC by 0.0653, from 0.7546 to 0.8199, compared to the factor-centered base case. A Wilcoxon test was performed on the 800 matched pairs of probabilistic prediction errors, generating an index of error reduction = 0.4575 and a normalized Z statistic = 11.14, with a two-tail p value < 0.00005.

5. Also in the training subsample, the PCM-based predictions improved AUC by 0.0367, from 0.7832 to 0.8199, compared to the practice-centered base case, which predicted solely on the basis of initial AJCC stage. A Wilcoxon test was performed on the 800 matched pairs of probabilistic prediction errors, generating an index of error reduction = 0.2125 and a normalized Z statistic = 4.19, with a two-tail p value < 0.00005.

Three prediction algorithms were generated from the 800-patient breast cancer training subsample in a similar manner.

1. The first algorithm produced individually tailored probabilities of experiencing MBC DEATH within five years of initial diagnosis. These probabilities constituted the factor-centered base case. They emerged from a standard (unstratified) logistic regression analysis of the five conventional prognostic factors used in breast cancer, wherein missing observations of each factor were replaced by the mean value of that factor in the 800-patient training subsample.

   Corresponding probabilities for the complete sample of 1,225 breast cancer patients were labeled N5YRDPR in section 4. The ROC curve associated with N5YRDPR probabilities was the lowest one in Figure 16.

   Factor-centered base case probabilities in the training subsample yielded an estimated AUC of 0.7363. AUC was estimated as 0.7433 for the factor-centered base case in the complete 1,225-patient sample.

2. The second algorithm produced similar probabilities based solely on a dummy-variable logistic regression analysis of AJCC stage at initial diagnosis. These probabilities constituted the practice-centered base case, wherein missing observations of AJCC stage at diagnosis were replaced as previously described for split-sample analysis.

   Corresponding probabilities for the complete sample of 1,225 breast cancer patients were labeled F5YRDPR in section 4. The ROC curve associated with F5YRDPR probabilities was the second-lowest one in Figure 16.

   Practice-centered base case probabilities in the training subsample yielded an estimated AUC of 0.7887. AUC was estimated as 0.8021 for the practice-centered base case in the complete 1,225-patient sample.

3. The third algorithm produced similar probabilities based on a composite logistic regression analysis stratified by AJCC stage at diagnosis (PCM). Missing observations of each factor were replaced by PCM as described in sections 2.5, 2.6, and 2.7.

   Corresponding probabilities for the complete sample of 1,225 breast cancer patients were labeled S5YRDPR in section 4. The ROC curve associated with S5YRDPR probabilities was the third-lowest one (second from the top) in Figure 16.

   PCM-generated probabilities in the training subsample yielded an estimated AUC of 0.8687. AUC was estimated as 0.8792 for PCM in the complete 1,225-patient sample.

4. In the training subsample, the PCM-based predictions improved AUC by 0.1324, from 0.7363 to 0.8687, compared to the factor-centered base case. A Wilcoxon test was performed on the 800 matched pairs of probabilistic prediction errors, generating an index of error reduction = 0.4875 and a normalized Z statistic = 13.94, with a two-tail p value < 0.00005.

5. Also in the training subsample, the PCM-based predictions improved AUC by 0.0800, from 0.7887 to 0.8687, compared to the practice-centered base case, which predicted solely on the basis of initial AJCC stage. A Wilcoxon test was performed on the 800 matched pairs of probabilistic prediction errors, generating an index of error reduction = 0.3400 and a normalized Z statistic = 9.38, with a two-tail p value < 0.00005.

Recall that the ultimate goal of split-sample reliability testing was to reproduce PCM's superior predictive accuracy in both validation subsamples. This was accomplished in the following manner.

1. The factor-centered prediction algorithm produced from the melanoma training subsample was applied to patients in the validation subsample. This yielded 422 MM DEATH probabilities with an estimated AUC of 0.7747.
2. The practice-centered prediction algorithm produced from the melanoma training subsample was also applied to patients in the validation subsample. This yielded a second set of 422 MM DEATH probabilities with an estimated AUC of 0.7902.
3. The composite, PCM-based prediction algorithm produced from the melanoma training subsample was also applied to patients in the

        validation subsample. This yielded a third set of 422 MM DEATH
        probabilities with an estimated AUC of 0.7980.

4. The 0.7980 - 0.7747 = 0.0233 improvement in AUC from the
   factor-centered to the PCM methodology was accompanied by an index of
   error reduction = 0.4123 and a Wilcoxon normalized Z statistic = 6.29,
   with a two-tail p value < 0.00005.

5. The 0.7980 - 0.7902 = 0.0078 improvement in AUC from the
   practice-centered to the PCM methodology was accompanied by an index of
   error reduction = 0.1943 and a Wilcoxon normalized Z statistic = 2.73,
   with a two-tail p value of 0.0063.

6. The factor-centered prediction algorithm produced from the breast
   cancer training subsample was applied to patients in the validation
   subsample. This yielded 425 MBC DEATH probabilities with an estimated
   AUC of 0.7631.

7. The practice-centered prediction algorithm produced from the breast
   cancer training subsample was also applied to patients in the
   validation subsample. This yielded a second set of 425 MBC DEATH
   probabilities with an estimated AUC of 0.8212.

8. The composite, PCM-based prediction algorithm produced from the breast
   cancer training subsample was also applied to patients in the
   validation subsample. This yielded a third set of 425 MBC DEATH
   probabilities with an estimated AUC of 0.8785.

9. The 0.8785 - 0.7631 = 0.1154 improvement in AUC from the
   factor-centered to the PCM methodology was accompanied by an index of
   error reduction = 0.5953 and a Wilcoxon normalized Z statistic = 11.20,
   with a two-tail p value < 0.00005.

10. The 0.8785 - 0.8212 = 0.0573 improvement in AUC from the
    practice-centered to the PCM methodology was accompanied by an index of
    error reduction = 0.3082 and a Wilcoxon normalized Z statistic = 6.36,
    with a two-tail p value < 0.00005.

Both split-sample reliability analyses were successful. Their results are
tabled on the following pages for easy reference.

In all tables, AUC stands for the estimated Area Under the Curve of a Receiver
Operating Characteristic (ROC) analysis. Areas are uniformly expressed as a
percentage of the maximum possible area. Higher area percentages indicate
greater prognostic accuracy.

In the last two rows of each table, the Index of Error Reduction, the Wilcoxon
Z value, and its accompanying P value refer to reductions in absolute
probabilistic error achieved relative to the prognostic methodology tabled in
the row of the table immediately above. Each index is constructed from and the
statistical test is applied to the matched pairs of individual probabilistic
prediction errors—one error in each matched pair being taken from the
methodology indicated by its row in the table, and the other error being taken
from the same patient's prediction via the alternative methodology indicated in
the row immediately above.

The Index of Error Reduction has been designed to mimic a correlation
coefficient. It is calculated as the net number of error reductions (i.e., the
number of reductions minus the number of increases) divided by the total number
of matched-pair comparisons. As a signed proportion, the index ranges in value
between -1.0 (when all comparisons generate error increases) and +1.0 (when all
comparisons generate error reductions). In the spirit of an ordinary
correlation coefficient, the error reduction index has a value of 0.0 when the
number of error reductions is exactly counterbalanced by an equal number of
error increases.

The distribution of differences between absolute probabilistic prediction errors can be quite skewed. It can also possess occasional outliers (extreme values). Because of this, differences calculated from matched pairs of absolute probabilistic prediction errors were tested by the Wilcoxon matched-pairs, signed-ranks test instead of by the more traditional matched-pairs T test. The T test would have assumed normally distributed error differences. The Wilcoxon test makes no distributional assumptions. The Wilcoxon test is also less sensitive to outliers. Compared to the T test, the Wilcoxon test has a relative efficiency (in its ability to reject the null hypothesis) near ninety-five percent for small samples and slightly better than ninety-five percent for very large samples. The Wilcoxon test produces exact one-tail and two-tail P values for sample sizes up to twenty-five. A normalized Z statistic corresponding to the Wilcoxon T statistic is calculated for sample sizes greater than twenty-five. The Z statistic is the Wilcoxon T statistic divided by its own standard deviation. The Z value is then referred to the unit normal distribution to obtain an appropriate P value.

Comparison of Predictive Accuracy Produced by Differing Prognostic
Methodologies for Melanoma Patients (Complete Sample: N = 1,222)

Prognostic Methodology	AUC	Index of Error Reduction	Wilcoxon Z Value	2-Tail P Value
Factor-Centered Base Case	76.24%	N/A	N/A	N/A
Practice-Centered Base Case	78.67%	0.3257	6.92	< 0.00005
Our PCM Methodology	82.08%	0.2128	6.28	< 0.00005

Notes:

1. The factor-centered base case methodology executed a standard (unstratified)
   logistic regression analysis of the six traditional prognostic factors
   defined by the AJCC, wherein missing observations of each factor were
   replaced by the mean value of that factor in the complete 1,222-patient
   melanoma sample.
2. The practice-centered base case methodology executed a dummy-variable
   logistic regression analysis of AJCC stage at initial diagnosis, with an
   extra "stage" added to account for all patients whose initial AJCC stage
   could not be determined.
3. Our PCM methodology first stratified patients into three separate risk
   subgroups according to their AJCC stage at initial diagnosis; then executed
   three separate logistic regressions of the six traditional prognostic
   factors defined by the AJCC, wherein missing observations of each factor
   were replaced as described in sections 2.5, 2.6, and 2.7; and then merged
   the prognostic algorithms generated by the three separate analyses into a
   single, composite algorithm as described in section 2.9.

Comparison of Predictive Accuracy Produced by Differing Prognostic
Methodologies for Melanoma Patients (Training Subsample: N = 800)

Prognostic Methodology	AUC	Index of Error Reduction	Wilcoxon Z Value	2-Tail P Value
Factor-Centered Base Case	75.46%	N/A	N/A	N/A
Practice-Centered Base Case	78.32%	0.2775	5.48	< 0.00005
Our PCM Methodology	81.99%	0.2125	4.19	< 0.00005

Notes:

1. The factor-centered base case methodology executed a standard (unstratified) logistic regression analysis of the six traditional prognostic factors defined by the AJCC, wherein missing observations of each factor were replaced by the mean value of that factor in the 800-patient melanoma training subsample.
2. The practice-centered base case methodology executed a dummy-variable logistic regression analysis of AJCC stage at initial diagnosis, with an extra "stage" added to account for all training patients whose initial AJCC stage could not be determined.
3. Our PCM methodology first stratified training patients into three separate risk subgroups according to their AJCC stage at initial diagnosis; then executed three separate logistic regressions of the six traditional prognostic factors defined by the AJCC, wherein missing observations of each factor were replaced as described in sections 2.5, 2.6, and 2.7; and then merged the prognostic algorithms generated by the three separate analyses into a single, composite algorithm as described in section 2.9.

Comparison of Predictive Accuracy Produced by Differing Prognostic
Methodologies for Melanoma Patients (Validation Subsample: N = 422)

Prognostic Methodology	AUC	Index of Error Reduction	Wilcoxon Z Value	2-Tail P Value
Factor-Centered Base Case	77.47%	N/A	N/A	N/A
Practice-Centered Base Case	79.02%	0.2464	4.27	< 0.00005
Our PCM Methodology	79.80%	0.1943	2.73	0.0063

Notes:

1. The three prediction algorithms produced from the 800-patient melanoma
   training subsample by the factor-centered base case methodology, the
   practice-centered base case methodology, and our PCM methodology were
   applied, separately, to the 422-patient melanoma validation subsample to
   generate the results in the three rows of the above table.
2. This table addresses directly the overfitting issue. Our PCM methodology
   produced a highly significant reduction in prediction errors relative both
   to the factor-centered base case and to the practice-centered base case
   methodologies. The significant error reductions occurred when a prediction
   algorithm fitted to the 800-patient melanoma training subsample was later
   applied to the 422-patient melanoma validation subsample. Achieving
   significantly improved prognostic accuracy relative to one set of patients
   cannot be attributed to overfitting a prediction algorithm to
   observations made on an entirely separate set of patients. The training and
   validation subsamples were completely distinct.

Comparison of Predictive Accuracy Produced by Differing Prognostic
Methodologies for Breast Cancer Patients (Complete Sample: N = 1,225)

Prognostic Methodology	AUC	Index of Error Reduction	Wilcoxon Z Value	2-Tail P Value
Factor-Centered Base Case	74.33%	N/A	N/A	N/A
Practice-Centered Base Case	80.21%	0.3143	7.57	< 0.00005
Our PCM Methodology	87.92%	0.3649	11.87	< 0.00005

Notes:

1. The factor-centered base case methodology executed a standard (unstratified) logistic regression analysis of the five conventional prognostic factors used in breast cancer, wherein missing observations of each factor were replaced by the mean value of that factor in the complete 1,225-patient breast cancer sample.
2. The practice-centered base case methodology executed a dummy-variable logistic regression analysis of AJCC stage at initial diagnosis, with an extra "stage" added to account for all patients whose initial AJCC stage could not be determined.
3. Our PCM methodology first stratified patients into three separate risk subgroups according to their AJCC stage at initial diagnosis; then executed three separate logistic regressions of the five conventional prognostic factors used in breast cancer, wherein missing observations of each factor were replaced as described in sections 2.5, 2.6, and 2.7; and then merged the prognostic algorithms generated by the three separate analyses into a single, composite algorithm as described in section 2.9.

Comparison of Predictive Accuracy Produced by Differing Prognostic
Methodologies for Breast Cancer Patients (Training Subsample: N = 800)

Prognostic Methodology	AUC	Index of Error Reduction	Wilcoxon Z Value	2-Tail P Value
Factor-Centered Base Case	73.63%	N/A	N/A	N/A
Practice-Centered Base Case	78.87%	0.2400	5.56	< 0.00005
Our PCM Methodology	86.87%	0.3400	9.38	< 0.00005

Notes:

1. The factor-centered base case methodology executed a standard (unstratified) logistic regression analysis of the five conventional prognostic factors used in breast cancer, wherein missing observations of each factor were replaced by the mean value of that factor in the 800-patient breast cancer training subsample.
2. The practice-centered base case methodology executed a dummy-variable logistic regression analysis of AJCC stage at initial diagnosis, with an extra "stage" added to account for all training patients whose initial AJCC stage could not be determined.
3. Our PCM methodology first stratified training patients into three separate risk subgroups according to their AJCC stage at initial diagnosis; then executed three separate logistic regressions of the five conventional prognostic factors used in breast cancer, wherein missing observations of each factor were replaced as described in sections 2.5, 2.6, and 2.7; and then merged the prognostic algorithms generated by the three separate analyses into a single, composite algorithm as described in section 2.9.

Comparison of Predictive Accuracy Produced by Differing Prognostic
Methodologies for Breast Cancer Patients (Validation Subsample: N = 425)

Prognostic Methodology	AUC	Index of Error Reduction	Wilcoxon Z Value	2-Tail P Value
Factor-Centered Base Case	76.31%	N/A	N/A	N/A
Practice-Centered Base Case	82.12%	0.3600	6.22	< 0.00005
Our PCM Methodology	87.85%	0.3082	6.36	< 0.00005

Notes:

1. The three prediction algorithms produced from the 800-patient breast cancer training subsample by the factor-centered base case methodology, the practice-centered base case methodology, and our PCM methodology were applied, separately, to the 425-patient breast cancer validation subsample to generate the results in the three rows of the above table.
2. This table addresses directly the overfitting issue. Our PCM methodology produced a highly significant reduction in prediction errors relative both to the factor-centered base case and to the practice-centered base case methodologies. The significant error reductions occurred when a prediction algorithm fitted to the 800-patient breast cancer training subsample was later applied to the 425-patient breast cancer validation subsample. Achieving significantly improved prognostic accuracy relative to one set of patients cannot be attributed to overfitting a prediction algorithm to observations made on an entirely separate set of patients. The training and validation subsamples were completely distinct.

ANNOTATED REFERENCES

1. Joensuu, Heikki, and Sakari Toikkanen. 1995. "Cured of Breast Cancer?" *Journal of Clinical Oncology* 13:62-69.

   This journal article documents the original analysis of the Turku data set. It also describes in detail how carefully the breast cancer data were collected and maintained.

2. Le, Chap T. 1997. *Applied Survival Analysis*. New York: John Wiley and Sons, Inc.

   This book provides an excellent introduction to and summary of many of the analytical and statistical procedures executed in the present book.

3. *STATVIEW Reference Manual* (Third edition). 1999. Cary, NC: SAS Institute, Inc.

   This reference manual and the accompanying user's manual were useful in validating for both logical and programming accuracy many of the procedures incorporated in the PCM methodology. Great care was taken to ensure that PCM procedures generated the same results as did STATVIEW when given the same input data to analyze.

4. Balch, Charles M. et al. 2001. "Prognostic Factors Analysis of 17,600 Melanoma Patients: Validation of the American Joint Committee on Cancer Melanoma Staging System." *Journal of Clinical Oncology* 19:3622-34.

   This journal article documents the analysis from which the anticipated five-year disease-specific survival probabilities by AJCC stage of disease progression were obtained, based on 17,600 melanoma patients. Section 3 of the present book describes how PCM divided our sample of 1,222 melanoma patients into risk groups that preserved the ranking of these anticipated survival probabilities.

5. Miller, James R. III. 2002. "A Bayesian Assessment of the Curative Impact of Medical Intervention." Stanford Business School Technical Report No. 86: Stanford, CA.

   This monograph introduces a conceptual framework and a collection of facilitating procedures to assess, probabilistically, both the curative impact of a specified medical intervention and the likelihood that a particular patient has been cured following that intervention.

   The logistic and Cox (proportional hazards) regression models are logically integrated by means of Bayes' theorem. Appropriately extended logistic regression supplies an individually tailored prior cure probability (prior to the intervention) for each patient. Appropriately extended Cox regression supplies an individually tailored conditional probability of survival time without further disease progression, if the patient remains at risk. Then, a Minimal Risk Partitioning Algorithm (MRPA) is constructed to assign an individually tailored posterior cure probability. It encapsulates the likelihood that each patient was actually cured following the intervention.

   MRPA also estimates a specified medical intervention's cure rate for any given patient population.

Individually tailored posterior cure probabilities are a function of the time elapsed since the intervention with no evidence of further disease progression. In this sense, they resemble survival probabilities—but with an all-important reversal in the direction of inference. A cure probability is defined as the conditional probability of having been cured (as opposed to remaining still at risk), given the duration of survival time free of further disease progression following some medical intervention. A survival probability is a reverse conditional probability. It indicates the likelihood of surviving for a specified period of time, given that the patient was not cured by the medical intervention and, therefore, remained still at risk following it and despite its curative potential.

It is through the application of Bayes' theorem that the direction of inference is successfully reversed. Reversing the direction of inference in this manner requires partitioning a set of patients who have undergone a potentially curative intervention into those who were and those who were not cured. This partitioning, in turn, reveals how failing to separate cured from noncured patients can sometimes lead to quite misleading conclusions. Performing a standard Kaplan-Meier survival analysis on a sample containing a substantial proportion of cured patients was shown to distort the stable hazard rate over time characterizing the noncured patients. Any traditional survival analysis performed on a nonpartitioned sample has the potential to give the false impression of a declining hazard rate.

In terms of methodological lineage, PCM is a direct descendant of MRPA. MRPA also begins by reconstructing conventional prognostic methodology to facilitate individual patient predictions. Both are designed to produce individually tailored focal event probabilities. In PCM, choice of the focal event is unrestricted. In MRPA, the focal event is always defined in terms of whether or not a particular patient has been transformed following a specified medical intervention from a prior state of being at risk to a posterior state of no longer remaining at substantial risk of further disease progression (i.e., to the state of now being cured).

Both PCM and MRPA were designed to exploit the facilities of and to execute within the same specialized software operating system (MDMS) employed and illustrated throughout this book. See particularly appendix A. Just like MRPA, PCM incorporates both the logistic and the Cox regression models. Because PCM selectively modifies both types of regression in exactly the manner required by MRPA it also enhances the ability of MRPA to produce more accurate cure probabilities.

6. Ware, James H. 2006. "The Limitations of Risk Factors as Prognostic Tools." *New England Journal of Medicine* 355:2615-17.

As described in section 1.2, this article by Dr. Ware in the *New England Journal of Medicine* served as the historical trigger for the development of PCM.

7. Kashani-Sabet, Mohammed, Richard W. Sagebiel, Heikki Joensuu, and James R. Miller III. 2013. "A Patient-Centered Methodology That Improves the Accuracy of Prognostic Predictions in Cancer." Published online February 2013 by *PLoS One*. http//www.plosone/article.0056435.

This journal article constitutes a condensed version of the present book introducing and explaining PCM. The condensed version was specifically designed to appeal to the community of practicing physicians.

INDEX

A

A5YRDPR attribute, 44–45, 53, 74–75
absolute probabilistic error, 14
adjuvant therapy, 79, 80–81
admissibility requirements, 17–18, 19, 24, 96
admissible cut point, 20
age of patient, 15, 64, 65, 75, 76f, 78, 92
AGEMUIRI, 39, 70
AJCC (American Joint Committee on Cancer), 14, 15
AJCC stage, 15, 17, 32, 33, 36–37, 40, 42, 43, 45, 50, 57, 63, 64, 65, 67, 70, 73, 91, 92, 94, 100
AJCC stage at diagnosis, 17, 31, 32, 33, 34, 38, 39, 43, 44, 50, 57, 64, 68, 69, 73, 74–75, 81, 92, 94
AJCC stage error, 32, 33
AJCC staging classification, 15, 17, 32, 38, 40, 42, 43, 50, 63, 68, 71, 72, 74, 79
AJCC T stage, 31
algorithms, 3, 6, 12–14, 18, 21, 25, 26, 36, 91, 92, 94, 95
altered focus, one of PCM's six differentiating characteristics, 5–6, 27
American Joint Committee on Cancer (AJCC), 14, 15
angiogenesis, 51, 57
ANOVA (randomized blocks two-way analysis of variance), 27–28, 32
assessment, of PCM, 26
AUC (Area Under the Curve), 14, 27

B

base case, establishing, 14–15
base case prognostic factors, 26
baseline hazard function, 13
baseline survival function, 13, 14
bilaterality, 79
binomial sign test, 27, 28, 29, 33
biomarkers, 4, 92
breast cancer patient sample
    applying PCM to, 63–89
    assessment of PCM for patients with, 26
    high-risk subgroup, 63, 70, 71, 75, 78
    low-risk subgroup, 63, 70, 71, 75, 78
    medium-risk subgroup, 63, 70, 71, 75, 78
    patients excluded from sample, 12
    patients in sample, 11
    prognostic factors, 15
    salient events in progression of, 10
    sample described, 63
    stratification by risk group, 63–65

summary of results, 83–89

C

CA5YRDPR attribute, 39, 69
California Pacific Medical Center (CPMC), v
Central Limit Theorem, 28
CF5YRDPR attribute, 37–38, 68
chi-square statistics, 45
circular reasoning, 99
Clark level of primary tumor invasion, 15, 45, 49f, 51
classical hypothesis testing, 98
CN5YRDPR attribute, 36, 67
conclusions/recommendations, 90–102
CONVAGE factor, 65, 71
conventions, statistical and presentational, 27
CONVMITC factor, 65, 71
CONVSITE factor, 65, 71
CONVSIZE factor, 65, 71
CONVULC factor, 65, 71
correct outcome prediction, rates of, 6
Cox regression analysis, 2, 4, 6, 11, 13, 14, 22, 23, 24, 25, 93
CPMC (California Pacific Medical Center), v
CS5YRDPR attribute, 39–40, 70
cut points, 14, 20, 21, 22, 84, 92
cutaneous melanoma, 31

D

data quality, 97
diagnosis, as highest-impact basis for stratification, 17
discrimination, 14, 18, 19, 53, 84
disease-specific death within five years, as common focal event, 11, 24, 31, 63
disease-specific survival (DSS), 12, 31, 34
dummy variables, 21, 22, 23, 32, 33. *See also* zero-one dummy variables

E

estrogen receptor (ER), 79
evidence-based perspective, iv, 1, 3
experience-based manner, iv

F

F5YRDPR attribute, 37–38, 43, 50, 53, 57, 58f, 68, 73, 78, 84, 86, 88f
factor weights, 25. *See also* weight (assigned to factors)
factor-centered
    as current paradigm, 1
    defined, iv
factor-centered base case
    and admissibility requirements, 18

with breast cancer patients, 15, 26, 83, 86, 100

with melanoma patients, 15, 26, 52, 57, 100

with missing observations, breast cancer, 71

with missing observations, melanoma, 40, 42, 43, 44

without missing observations, breast cancer, 65, 68, 69, 72, 74, 75

without missing observations, melanoma, 34, 36, 38, 39

Finland, breast cancer data set from, v, 63, 97

fitted relationships, 18

five-year outcomes, 12

FN1, 51, 57

focal end point/focal event, 10-13, 16, 18, 21, 22, 31, 63

focal prediction, 16

focal question, 90-92, 94, 96

follow-up, 12, 31, 63, 97, 101

formal hypothesis tests, 5, 28

Friedman two-way analysis of variance by ranks, 28, 32, 33

G

G15YRDPR attribute, 52, 53, 80, 84

G25YRDPR attribute, 52-55, 56*f*, 57, 58*f*, 59, 80, 83-86, 87*f*, 88*f*

gene expression, degrees of, 51

generalizable research conclusions, 2

goodness-of-fit improvement, 92-93

H

hazard function, 13

hazard ratios, 2, 5, 23, 24, 93

HER2, 63

heterogeneity, 16, 17, 57, 89

high-dose alpha-2b interferon (IFN), 59

higher subscale, 20

high-risk subgroup
breast cancer patients, 63, 70, 71, 75, 78
melanoma, 34, 35*f*, 39, 40, 45

historical trigger, 5

homogeneity, 16, 17, 57, 89

hypothesis testing, 98

hypothetical procedure, appearing to improve predictive accuracy, 95-96

I

IFN (high-dose alpha-2b interferon), 59

impact-reflecting indexes, 21-24

inadmissible observations, 13

incidence rank order, 34

incorporating additional factors, one of PCM's six differentiating characteristics, 8-9

index of error reduction, 29, 33, 38, 39, 40, 43, 44, 45, 50, 52, 53, 68, 69, 71, 74, 75, 78, 80, 83, 100, 101

individually tailored probabilities, 12-14, 27, 37, 54, 59, 67, 84, 85, 86. *See also* tailored individual probabilities

inflammatory cancer, 79

K

Kaplan-Meier analysis, 7, 11, 22, 34, 35*f*, 59, 60*f*, 61*f*, 62*f*, 65, 66*f*, 81, 82*f*, 93

Kendall rank correlation test, 29

Kruskal-Wallis test, 29, 34, 65

L

least-squares weights, 25

"The Limitations of Risk Factors as Prognostic Tools" (Ware), 4

logistic regression analysis, 2, 6, 11, 12, 13, 21, 22, 24, 25

lower subscale, 20

low-risk subgroup
breast cancer patients, 63, 70, 71, 75, 78
melanoma, 34, 35*f*, 39, 40, 45

M

M (metastasis) scale, 79

Mann-Whitney test, 19, 29, 34

matched-pair comparisons, 29

matched-pairs T test, 27, 28, 33

matched-sample comparisons, 27

MBC death, 63, 64, 67, 75, 78, 79, 81, 84, 85, 86, 100, 101

mean probability, 14

medicine
as art, iv, v, 3
as science, iv, v

medium-risk subgroup
breast cancer patients, 63, 70, 71, 75, 78
melanoma, 34, 35*f*, 39, 40, 45

melanoma patient sample
applying PCM to, 31-62
assessment of PCM for patients with, 26
high-risk subgroup, 34, 35*f*, 39, 40, 45
low-risk subgroup, 34, 35*f*, 39, 40, 45
medium-risk subgroup, 34, 35*f*, 39, 40, 45
patients excluded from sample, 12
patients in sample, 11, 31
prognostic factors, 14-15
salient events in progression of, 10
staging classification, 15

subsets in terms of G25YRDPR
    probabilities, 59
summary of results, 52–58
microsatellites, 51
missing observations
    analysis of traditional prognostic
        factors with, breast cancer, 71–79
    analysis of traditional prognostic
        factors with, melanoma, 40–51
    analysis of traditional prognostic
        factors without, breast cancer,
        65–71
    analysis of traditional prognostic
        factors without, melanoma, 32–34
    collected into training subsample, 22
    dealing with as one of PCM's six
        differentiating characteristics, 8
    as handled separately across
        heterogeneous strata, 7
    SPSA algorithm assigns particular
        numeric values to, 29
    SPSA algorithm dealing with, 93
missing patient data, 29
mitotic count, 63, 64, 79, 89
mitotic rate, 8, 15, 22, 24, 32, 33, 36, 45,
    48f, 57, 75, 92
MM death, 31, 32, 33, 34, 36, 37, 45, 50,
    51, 54, 55, 59, 75, 100
molecular factors, 51, 52
multivariate statistical analysis, 17, 32

N

N (nodal involvement) scale, 79
N5YRDPR attribute, 41, 50, 53, 57, 58f, 72,
    78, 84, 86, 88f
natural logarithms, 24
necrosis, degree of, 79
New England Journal of Medicine, 4–5, 90
nonmissing observations, 22
nonparametric statistical tests, 29–30, 32
non-population-based scholarship, 92
nontraditional prognostic factors
    addition of to traditional factors,
        breast cancer, 79–80, 83
    addition of to traditional factors,
        melanoma, 51–52
    impact of addition of to base case, 26
    predicting MBC death, list of in two
        groups, 79–80
    predicting MM death, list of in two
        groups, 51
    and predictive accuracy, 31
    search for new, 101, 102
novel success measures, 5, 27–30
nuclear pleomorphism, degree of, 79

O

outliers, 28, 29, 32, 33

overall survival (OS), 12
overfitting, 7, 18, 30, 92–97, 99, 100

P

p values, 5
parametric statistical tests, 29–30
partitioning procedure, 18–21
patient age, 15, 45, 46f, 64, 65, 75,
    76f, 92
patient attribute/index, 22
patient follow-up, 12. *See also* follow-up
patient sex, 15, 40, 45, 65, 92
patient-centered
    defined, v, 90
    as extension of factor-centered, 1, 98
    transition to as reoriented paradigm
        enhancement, 4
Patient-Centered Methodology (PCM)
    ability to incorporate nontraditional
        and nonconventional prognostic
        factors, 99
    compared to traditional prognostic
        methodology, 5–9
    degrees of freedom, 96
    goals/objectives of, 5, 27, 99
    as identifying high-risk patients
        significantly more reliably for IFN
        treatment, 59
    interpretations of, 94
    "The Limitations of Risk Factors as
        Prognostic Tools" as historical
        trigger for development of, 5
    novel procedural devices in, 90–91
    reason for dividing prognostic factors
        into separate groups using, 51
    in ten steps, 1–2
PHIP, 51, 57
population-based scholarship, 16, 90
positive lymph nodes, number of, 51
practice-centered base case
    breast cancer summary, 83, 86
    melanoma summary, 53, 57
    with missing observations, breast
        cancer, 71, 72, 75, 78
    with missing observations, melanoma,
        42, 45
    without missing observations, breast
        cancer, 67, 68, 69
    without missing observations, melanoma,
        37, 39
"precleaning" of data, 97
prediction errors, 28, 32, 33, 40, 55, 85,
    86, 96
predictions of events, 11
predictive accuracy
    of G25YRDPR composite probability, 87f
    improved by increasing size of training
        sample, 18

168

improvements in, v, 4, 5–6, 31, 39, 40,
45, 50, 52–53, 70, 75, 78, 83, 93,
100–101
measures of, 14, 27
relative (univariate), 33
scattergram of, G25YRDPR composite
probability, breast cancer, 87*f*
scattergram of, G25YRDPR composite
probability, melanoma, 56*f*
predictive relationships, iv, 2, 3, 96
predictive scale characteristics, 6
preprocessing, 24, 25, 92
probabilistic prediction errors, 6, 28, 32,
33, 40
probabilistic predictions, 5, 27, 29, 37,
40, 50, 53, 54, 67, 71, 79, 84, 94, 104
progesterone receptor (PR), 79
prognostic factors
as basis for making individually
tailored predictions, v
as dichotomous, 8, 45, 75, 92
generalizability of, 2
indicator as called, iv
prognostic modeling, 3
prognostic research, purpose of, iv
proportional hazards model, 23
proportional weighting procedure, 93

R

radiation therapy, 79, 81, 89
randomized blocks two-way analysis of
variance (ANOVA), 27–28, 32
raw measurement scale, 17–24, 92
recommendations/conclusions, 90–102
relative (multivariate) statistical
significance, 33
relative (univariate) predictive
accuracy, 33
relative predictive potency weights, 57,
89, 94
relative prognostic potency, 24
replication, 99–102
risk groups, merging of, 25–26
risk subgroups, 31–34, 39, 40, 42, 43, 45,
50, 52, 57, 63–65, 70–71, 75, 78, 80,
81, 89, 97
ROC (Receiver-Operating-Characteristic), 27
ROC analyses, 58*f*, 88*f*
ROC/AUC analysis, 11, 14, 27
ROC/AUC scores, 6

S

S5YRDPR attribute, 45, 50, 52, 53, 57, 58*f*,
78, 80, 84, 86, 88*f*
salient end points, 17
sample size, 93, 95, 97

Scale Partitioning and Spacing Algorithm
(SPSA), 7, 18, 21, 26, 30, 36, 38, 50,
92, 98
scale partitions, 21
scattergrams
of predictive accuracy of G25HYRDPR
composite probability, melanoma,
56*f*
of predictive accuracy of G25YRDPR
composite probability, breast
cancer, 87*f*
of UIRI for age at initial diagnosis,
breast cancer, 76*f*
of UIRI for age at initial diagnosis,
melanoma, 46*f*
of UIRI for Clark level of primary
tumor, melanoma, 49*f*
of UIRI for mitotic rate of primary
tumor, melanoma, 48*f*
of UIRI for size of primary tumor,
breast cancer, 77*f*
of UIRI for thickness of primary tumor,
melanoma, 47*f*
selection bias, 80–81
selective focus, one of PCM's six
differentiating characteristics, 6
selective stratification, one of PCM's six
differentiating characteristics, 6–7
sex of patient, 15, 40, 45, 65, 92
similar-segment-based sample, 16
Spearman rank correlation test, 29
split-sample analyses, 100
SPSA conversion, one of PCM's six
differentiating characteristics,
7–8. *See also* Scale Partitioning and
Spacing Algorithm (SPSA)
staging classification, 15, 17. *See also*
AJCC staging classification
standard index, 91
statistical significance, 1, 29, 32, 33, 99
statistical tests, 27–28
stratification
according to risk of experiencing focal
event, 16–17
factors that are candidates for, 91
impact of, 91, 93, 95
requirements for, 92
stratification by risk group
both training samples, 25, 97
breast cancer patients, 63, 64–65, 70,
71, 75
melanoma patients, 32–34, 40
preprocessing steps, 24
stratification variable, 91
stratifying attribute/index, 22
subsamples, 18–23, 25, 95, 96, 99–101
subscale partition size, 22
subscales, 7, 19, 20–24, 54–55, 85–86

sub-subsamples, 22
sub-subscales, 22
survival probability, 14

T

T (tumor characteristic) scale, 79
tailored individual probabilities, 14,
    59-62. *See also* individually tailored
    probabilities
Tamoxifen, 80-81
ten-year outcomes, 12
therapeutic choices, applying tailored
    individual probabilities to, 59-62
tied observations, 29
tied prediction error differences, 32
TIL (tumor-infiltrating lymphocytes)
    level, 51
total-population-based sample, 16
traditional prognostic factors
    analysis of with missing observations,
        melanoma, 40-50
    analysis of without missing
        observations, melanoma, 34-40
    in breast cancer, 63
    diverse impact of, 45
traditional prognostic research/analysis
    compared to PCM, 5-9
    focus of, 2
    patient population in, 4
    as performed before using base case
        prognostic factors, 26
training data, 92, 96
training samples, 3, 5-8, 18--25, 94, 97
training subsamples, 25, 100
tubule formation, extent of, 79
tumor grade, 63, 79, 89
tumor histological subtype, 51, 79
tumor regression, degree of, 51
tumor size, 63, 64, 75, 77*f*
tumor thickness, 31, 32, 33, 45, 47*f*, 57,
    75, 92
tumor vascularity, 51
tumor-infiltrating lymphocytes (TIL)
    level, 51
Turku data set, 63, 75, 80, 89
two-tail tests, 28

U

ULCHUIRI, 70
ULCLUIRI, 70
ULCMUIRI, 70
unavailable observations, 22
uniform null hypothesis, 28
United States Weather Bureau, 54
univariate discriminability, 18-21
Univariate Impact-Reflecting Index (UIRI),
    7, 20, 21-25, 32, 36, 38, 39, 40, 46*f*,
    71, 76*f*, 77*f*, 92, 93, 98

University of California San Francisco
    (UCSF), v, 31, 97

V

validation procedure, 99
validation subsamples, 99, 100, 101
vascular involvement, 51, 57

W

Ware, James H., 4-5, 8, 10, 11, 14, 27, 32,
    33, 53, 83, 90, 99
weight (assigned to factors), 25, 57, 89,
    93, 94
weighted average biomarker score, 4
weighting UIRI values, 24-25
Wilcoxon matched-pairs, signed-ranks test,
    27, 28, 29, 33, 39, 40
within-pair tied observations, 29
within-risk-subgroup, 51

Z

zero-one dummy variables, 21, 23, 37, 42,
    43, 67, 68, 73

AUTHOR BIOGRAPHIES

For more than thirty years James R. Miller III, PhD, was a professor at the Stanford Graduate School of Business. He has been doing full-time cancer research since his retirement in 1997 as Walter and Elise Haas Professor of Business Administration. He received a Bachelors Degree from Princeton University, a Woodrow Wilson Fellowship (University of California at Berkeley), an MBA from the Harvard Business School, and a PhD from the Massachusetts Institute of Technology. He has previously published a book, Professional Decision Making, and more than 40 monographs and articles in professional journals. Professor Miller is the author of six software patents. He has served on more than a dozen Boards of Directors in the United States and Europe and as CEO of two start-up companies in the Silicon Valley. He has three daughters and six grandchildren.

Mohammed Kashani-Sabet, MD, is Medical Director of Cancer Programs at the California Pacific Medical Center (CPMC). He also serves as director of the Center for Melanoma Research and Treatment and senior scientist at the CPMC Research Institute. Dr. Kashani-Sabet earned his medical degree from the State University of New York at Stony Brook, where he also completed an internship in internal medicine. He then completed a residency in dermatology at the University of California, San Francisco (UCSF), as well as a post-doctoral fellowship in cutaneous oncology, and received training in both dermatology and medical oncology. Dr. Kashani-Sabet maintains clinical interests in melanoma and cutaneous lymphoma, and research interests in targeted therapy, ribozymes, siRNAs, tumor metastasis, prognostic factors, and tumor biomarkers.

Richard W. Sagebiel, MD, was born in Ohio in 1934. He received his Bachelor's Degree from Yale University in 1956 in Music and Literature. He did his medical studies at the Harvard Medical School, including a year of pathology and research between his second and third years at the Massachusetts General Hospital (MGH). After an intern year of general medicine, he returned to MGH to study Dermatopathology with Wallace H. Clark, MD. He completed his training in the Departments of Dermatology and Pathology at the University of Washington Medical School. In 1970, he joined the Clinical Faculty of the University of California at San Francisco (UCSF), working with M. Scott Blois, PhD, MD, and others to form a clinical cooperative Melanoma Group. This group included Drs. Clark, Fitzpatrick (Harvard), and Kopf (NYU), and it stimulated the creation of other Melanoma Groups throughout the country. From 1988 to 1998, he was Director of the UCSF Melanoma Clinic. He then retired and became a Consulting Pathologist to that clinic.